THE POLYAMORISTS
NEXT DOOR

THE POLYAMORISTS NEXT DOOR

Inside Multiple-Partner Relationships and Families

Elisabeth Sheff

ROWMAN & LITTLEFIELD PUBLISHERS, INC.
Lanham • Boulder • New York • Toronto • Plymouth, UK

Rowman & Littlefield
4501 Forbes Boulevard, Suite 200, Lanham, Maryland 20706
www.rowman.com

10 Thornbury Road, Plymouth PL6 7PP, United Kingdom

British Library Cataloguing in Publication Information Available

Library of Congress Cataloging-in-Publication Data
Sheff, Elisabeth, 1969–
The polyamorists next door : inside multiple-partner relationships and families / Elisabeth Sheff.
pages cm
Includes bibliographical references and index.
ISBN 978-1-4422-2295-3 (cloth : alk. paper)—ISBN 978-1-4422-2296-0 (electronic)
1. Non-monogamous relationships. 2. Open marriage. 3. Families. 4. Sexual ethics. I. Title.
HQ980.A527 2010
306.84—dc23
2013024916

∞™ The paper used in this publication meets the minimum requirements of
American National Standard for Information Sciences Permanence of Paper
for Printed Library Materials, ANSI/NISO Z39.48-1992.

Printed in the United States of America

CONTENTS

ACKNOWLEDGMENTS

I would like to thank the following people and organizations for their support across the many years I have conducted the Polyamorous Families study and written this book. This book would not have been possible without all of you.

Patricia and Peter Adler; Serena Anderlini-D'Onofrio; the American Association of Sexuality Educators, Counselors, and Therapists (AASECT); Meg Barker; Jonathan, Jordan, Mike, and Tess Berger; Francesca Coin; the Community Academic Alliance for Research on Alternative Sexualities (CARAS); Stephanie Coontz; Dawn Davidson; Kris DeWelde; Denise Donnelly; Shari Dworkin; Maureen Ewell; Alice Fothergill; Terry Gross; Rhett Gayle; Corie Hammers; Ken Haslam; David LaPorta; Ryam Nearing; Maria Pallotta-Chiarolli; Erika Pluhar; Polyfamilies; PolyResearchers; Adina Nack; Donald Reitzes; Erin Ruel; Christine, Colby, Elaine, and Jonathan Sheff; Wendy Simonds; Suzanne Staszak-Silva; Sociologists for Women in Society (SWS); the Society for the Study of Social Problems (SSSP); Cascade and Zhahai Spring; Tristan Taormino; Geraldine Thompson; Robyn Trask; Chandra Ward; Mary Wolf; and the many participants who allowed me to ask them probing questions about their families—thanks for your time and your candor!

INTRODUCTION

"Ahhh, that was great! I was starved," Dani Warren said, pushing back from the table. In her mid-forties, white, highly educated, middle class, and liberal, Dani looked every inch the poly hippie mom. Next to her sat Lex, one of her husbands, and next to him sat Mike, their mutual husband and third member in the Warren triad. Lex had whipped up a Mexi-Cali feast that the four adults and four children seated around the table had just devoured, and we sat chatting before clearing the table. Mike commented, "The rice was excellent, just the right amount of spice. Thanks for making dinner, Lex." Lex responded "Eli helped. She was my sous Sheff. Get it? Sous chef?" Chuckling over the pun they had made with my last name, the two men smiled at each other and touched hands. "Well thanks to you, too, then, Eli," Mike responded.

❉ ❉ ❉ ❉ ❉

In this book you will meet families like the Warrens, who are polyamorous. They are your bankers, information technology specialists, teachers, and dentists. Like your other neighbors, they love their children, still owe on their student loans, forget to floss, and could probably stand to lose a few pounds. The thing that sets them apart from your other neighbors is that they have (or are open to having) multiple romantic partners at the same time and with each other's consent.

Polyamory is not for everyone. Complex, time-consuming, and potentially fraught with emotional booby traps, polyamory is tremendously rewarding for some people and a complete disaster for others. While I explain it in far greater detail later in the book, here I briefly define *polyamory* as consensual and emotionally intimate nonmonogamous relationships in which both women and men can negotiate to have multiple partners.

This book reports the results of my fifteen-year ethnographic study of polyamorous families with children.[1] I quote these poly folks throughout the book, using pseudonyms for everyone. People with first and last names are members of families I know well, usually because I interviewed them several times over the years and often interviewed many of their family members. People who only have first names are people I know less about because I only interviewed them once or chatted with them at a social event or online.[2] Because I quote many people, and it can be a little confusing, I have included a list in Appendix A of the families I frequently refer to for clarity. There is also Appendix B with more information on my research methods.

Initially, I approached polyamory as a "civilian" rather than a researcher. I was madly in love with a man who wanted to be nonmonogamous, and as an intellectual I try to understand things that frighten me. I was terrified of nonmonogamy, or what I learned in 1995 was called *polyamory* when I heard a National Public Radio interview with Ryam Nearing, then publisher of the polyamorous magazine *Loving More*.[3] In an effort to master my fear, I sought out the local poly community and began asking members how they managed their multiple-partner relationships. Deep into the graduate school process by then, it eventually became clear to me that the social implications of such an unconventional relationship style would make an ideal dissertation, so I formalized my initial self-serving questions into an official study with the university's Institutional Research Board (IRB) approval in 1996. Sixteen years later, I am almost fully recovered from my near brush with polyamory that drove me to sell my house and move to a different state to run away from disaster, and which expanded my mind, broke my heart, and ended my fifteen-year romantic relationship.

While I do not identify as polyamorous myself, I see it as a legitimate relationship style that can be tremendously rewarding for adults and provide excellent nurturing for children. Most of the evidence I use in this book comes from the many wonderful people who volunteered their time and energy to participate in interviews, though I also include some of my own experiences in chapter 4 because they are emblematic of what can happen when poly relationships go awry.

Polyamorous families are increasingly common, though fairly little is known about them outside of their own social circles. This book provides the information for people who wish to understand these complex and unusual relationships that are springing up across the United States, Canada, Europe, and Australia. As these families spread, professionals from counselors and therapists or educators and clergy to medical staff and lawyers will need factual information based in sound research to help them serve this growing client base.

CONTEMPORARY FAMILIES

Popular opinion among social conservatives in the United States harkens back to an idyllic 1950s family as the ideal familial form, portraying current society as floundering in a state of decay and lamenting a perceived loss or dilution of "the family"—a heterosexual, monogamous, legally married, two-parent, procreational unit that provides children with stable home environments run by a wage-earning father and supported by a mother who is a full-time parent.[4] In truth, families have always been in transition, and shifts toward single-parent and remarried families both cause and are affected by changes in labor markets and other social institutions.[5] The current cultural fascination in the United States with an idyllic vision of "traditional marriage" reinforces a romanticized, patriarchal family that never existed as we pretend it did. Pretending families used to be static institutions that never evolved and only began to change with the sexual revolution of the 1960s creates the false impression that families today are caught in an unprecedented state of chaos.

While "the" family has never been a static institution, changes in family life in the United States accelerated dramatically during the second half of the twentieth century. Most significantly, middle-class women entered the paid workforce en masse, precipitating dramatic shifts in gender norms and marital relationships.[6] Two especially important trends have been the rise in divorce and the subsequent creation of "blended families"[7] and serial monogamy, and the increase in single parenthood through divorce[8] and nonmarital childbirth.[9] For some, this move toward disengaging marriage from traditional gender roles and childbearing restrictions has opened fresh family possibilities, creating new options for people in same-sex relationships,[10] women who become pregnant through donor insemination,[11] and nonmonogamists.

Nonmonogamies

During the 1970s, academic researchers studied nonmonogamous relationships such as swinging,[12] mate swapping,[13] and open marriage,[14] focusing almost exclusively on open relationships among heterosexual white people. Research on sexually nonexclusive relationships dwindled in the 1980s, as the sexual revolution collided with the spread of the AIDS epidemic and a backlash of political conservatism.[15] It was during this period of social and political turmoil that polyamory emerged as an identity and a familial form.

While polyamorists have written about their relationships and familial experiences,[16] outside of my own research that explains polyamorous parenting strategies[17] and examines the "slippery slope" between same-sex marriage and polyamory,[18] few scholars have studied polyamorous families. Rubin briefly mentions polyamory in his review of family studies in which he documents a decline in the study of nonmonogamous relationships.[19] Bettinger uses a family systems approach to introduce factors that impact a "stable and high functioning gay male polyamorous family" of seven people—five adults and their two teen-aged sons.[20] Using examples from lesbian, gay, and poly families, Riggs explores various possibilities for kinship structures that value children's definitions of and contributions to their families, rather than relying solely on the adults' views of the relationships.[21] Pallotta-Chiarolli examines polyamorous relationships among women and their actively bisexual husbands,[22] and "polyfamilies'" interactions with school systems, detailing the costs of invisibility[23] and the strategies these families use to manage their interactions with school personnel and bureaucracies.[24] In her most recent book, Pallotta-Chiarolli investigates the state of "border families" composed of bisexual members, those in "mixed-orientation" marriages (gay/straight, poly/mono), and polyamorous families with children, concluding that educational programs designed for gay relationships do not sufficiently address issues specific to bisexual or polyamorous students and families.[25]

Serial Monogamy

The contemporary social reality is that families are changing—very few people in the general population expect to be monogamous in the classical sense of marrying as a virgin and having one sexual partner for their entire lifetimes. Rather, most people establish a monogamous relationship for a period of time with one person, break up,[26] and establish another monogamous relationship with someone else—a cycle called *serial monogamy*. As a consequence, a growing number of people in the United States today have children with one person and then create another family later with another person, thus involving multiple adults in the lives of children. These social shifts make it increasingly important to understand the fluidity of sexuality and families as well, and this research can be instrumental in translating research findings from polyamorous families to educational materials and policies useful to remarried and blended families with multiple adults in monogamous relationships responsible for children.

Family Resilience

Studies of family resilience emphasize a strengths-based perspective, examining the ways in which families deal with crises and develop adaptive behaviors to navigate the effects of adverse life events.[27] People who study resilient families seek to identify risks and protective mechanisms that help people through adversity, as well as tracking the strategies these families use as they attempt to balance risks with capabilities.[28] Resilient families are in a constant process of creation and recreation as they adapt to changing circumstances, and researchers have identified a number of protective processes that shield families in crises.[29] Two important protective processes are family cohesiveness, or the "balance between family separateness and connectedness," and the degree of flexibility, or the "balance between change and stability."[30] With their extensive communication and habit of tailoring their relationships to suit their needs, we shall see that the polyamorous families in this book generally have high levels of connectedness, flexibility, and resilience.

EVOLUTION OF THE TERM *POLYAMORY*

The word *polyamory* has a rich background. People involved in multiple-partner relationships in the 1960s, 1970s, and early 1980s sought words to express their ideas, found Standard English lacking, and began to create their own words. While the term *polyamory* was certainly coined by a member of the polyamorous community, exactly which person created the term is a matter of contention. One version claims the word *polyamory* is an outgrowth of the term *polyfidelity*, which Judson "Bro" Jud of the Kerista group had coined to mean "faithful to many."[31] Kerista, a polyamorous commune based in San Francisco that existed from 1971 to 1991, was an important element in founding the polyamorous community in the Bay Area and then nationwide. Jud, cofounder of Kerista with Even Eve, intended the term *polyfidelity* to mean, as a longtime Keristan told me, "closed and committed family units of up to a dozen bonded lovers, sexually faithful (exclusive) with each other."[32] Enacting this ideal for Keristans included creating an "equitable" sleeping schedule in which partners rotated nightly. Officially, Keristans were not to engage in same-sex lovemaking, though this rule was not always observed in practice.

"Janea," a woman who lived at Kerista for a number of years, credits Geo Barnes of Kerista with coining the term *polyfidelity* during a group discussion. "They were looking for something positive to say rather than use the frequently used 'non-monogamous' term." Janea remembers that the initial term *polyfidelity* branched to the more inclusive *polyamory* when Morning Glory Zell-Ravenheart,[33] the "senior wife" of the foundational Ravenheart clan with Oberon Zell-Ravenheart[34]

> came up with the term in the early nineties . . . in reaction to the fact that Kerista coined polyfidelity and it included sexual fidelity to your group—many who were interested in being poly did not want fidelity as part of the form, so they used polyfidelity to describe themselves even if they weren't. This created discord in the community and infighting about what is fidelity, etc. So Morning Glory was part of the group searching for another umbrella term that would include those who wanted to be poly and love their partners, but could include those with or without any agreement to fidelity within a closed circle of lovers.

The Ravenheart website cites the first appearance of the term *poly-amory* in Morning Glory's foundational "A Bouquet of Lovers" (also referred to as "Rules of the Road"), which appeared in an article in *Green Egg*, a Ravenheart Church of All Worlds publication. Morning Glory was searching for "a simple term to express the idea of having multiple simultaneous sexual/loving relationships without necessarily marrying everyone" and coined the term *polyamory* to be both an ex-pression of the lifestyle and a more positive way to express what practi-tioners had previously labeled *responsible nonmonogamy*, a term that had contentiously evolved into *polyfidelity*. The Ravenheart clan also contributed the term *monamory* or "love of one" to the polyamorous lexicon to provide an alternative to the cultural conception that monog-amy fit all occasions, when in current usage it customarily refers to steady dating rather than simply marriage to one other person.

OVERVIEW OF THE BOOK

The book is divided in to three parts. Part I, Understanding Polyamor-ous Relationships, provides an overview of the relationship style and communities. Chapter 1 defines polyamory and explains the different types of poly relationships, levels of emotional intimacy, and key terms. Chapter 2 explores who does polyamory and why, including demo-graphic characteristics of sample and community members, common rules that structure poly relationships, and the motivations people re-port for establishing poly relationships. Polyamorous communities are the focus of chapter 3, including a brief history of nonmonogamy, the overlap with other communities, and some characteristics of poly com-munities. Chapter 4 explains issues facing poly relationships, such as jealousy, sexually transmitted infections, and dealing with stigma.

Part II focuses on polyamorous families with children. Chapter 5 explains how children in polyamorous families fare, and chapter 6 fo-cuses on adults in poly families. Using data from adults and children, chapter 7 explains the benefits to poly family life, such as added re-sources, emotional intimacy, expanding family support, and being open-minded. Chapter 8 explores the down side of poly families, examining issues such as partners leaving, stigma, and family friction. It is impor-tant to note that the disadvantages poly families deal with are the same ones facing serial monogamous families, and that these difficulties are not distinctive to polyamorous families. In chapter 9, poly people reveal the strategies parents and kids use to deal with the disadvantages, such as emotional protection, stigma management, and creating chosen family.

Part III, Conclusions, takes the information from the study and examines how it can be useful to the many people who do not identify as polyamorous. Chapter 10 details the ideas and strategies that poly people use to navigate their complex relationships and the ways in which these techniques can be useful for people in monogamous relationships and families, as well as the policy implications this research indicates.

Part One

Understanding Polyamorous Relationships

I

WHAT IS POLYAMORY?

Polyamory is consensual, openly conducted, multiple-partner relationships in which both men and women have negotiated access to additional partners outside of the traditional committed couple. It is not *polygamy* (marriage of many) because polyamorists are not always married. Even more importantly, polygamy is almost always practiced as *polygyny*, or one man married to multiple women. Usually in those relationships, the women are not allowed to have additional male partners and are prohibited from having sex with each other. Polyamory is also not *cheating* because (ideally) everyone is aware of the other partners—the relationships have been negotiated with rules to structure scheduling and safer-sex agreements. It is also not *swinging*, which tends to be more focused on sexual variety and less accepting of emotional intimacy. Some swingers in fact negotiate arrangements that prohibit emotional connection or even repeated interaction with the same lover. Polyamory can also overlap with the versions of swinging that allow emotional intimacy, and the intersection between polyamory and swinging is common enough that Ken Haslam (a well-known polyamory activist) coined the term *swolly* to describe the juncture between the two relationship styles. Chapter 3 discusses the intersection of polyamory and swinging in greater detail.

The gender equality that exists (at least ideally) between women and men distinguishes polyamory from many other forms of nonmonogamies,[1] and this has important implications for where polyamory occurs in the world. Most popular in Australia, Canada, the United States, and

Western Europe, polyamory only flourishes where women can be the social equal of the men around them. For many of my respondents, this translated to women actively pursuing the education and professional skills that allowed them to be financially self-sufficient, with or without male partners.

QUICK FACTS ABOUT POLYAMOROUS PEOPLE

People who have polyamorous relationships are called *polyamorists*, and they use the term *poly* as a noun (a person who is poly engages in polyamorous relationships), an adjective (to describe something that has polyamorous qualities), and an umbrella term that includes polyfidelity, or relationships based in sexual and emotional fidelity among a group larger than a dyad. Some poly people are legally married, and others span a wide range of types and levels of commitment. Some live together, usually in groups of two to five, and others live alone or with roommates. Many have children, some of them from previous monogamous relationships, and others are born into poly households.

Many people in poly communities have a suspicion of institutions and a rebellious streak.[2] This can translate into a rejection of conventional relationships with institutions and a willingness to exist outside of institutions that most take for granted, such as homeschooling and homebirth. In line with this suspicion of institutions, most of my respondents did not practice any religion, but significant minorities were Pagan or Unitarian Universalist, with a smattering of Jews, Buddhists, and Christians. Like other sexual minorities, poly people tend to live in cities or suburban areas where it is easier to meet potential partners and have more privacy than it is in many small towns or rural areas. The polyamorists who have participated in research (mine and other's[3]) tend to be white, well-educated, liberal, and middle to upper-middle class.

Unfortunately, there are no reliable statistics about the number of polyamorous people. Like other sexual minorities, people with poly relationships tend to be closeted because being openly poly, gay, kinky, or otherwise sexually unconventional can have serious consequences, such as the loss of jobs, friends, family, housing, and custody of children. Further complicating the question of the number of poly people is that it is difficult to decide whom to include in the count. Should it include everyone who is in an openly conducted, nonmonogamous relationship, regardless of the boundaries that structure their relationships? Only the people who identify as polyamorous and interact with poly communities? Even with the difficulties inherent in identifying the population, folks on poly Internet sites estimate that between 1.2 and 9.8 million people in the United States are polyamorous and/or nonmonogamous.

Polyamorists hope to create a variety of relationships—both long and short term—that are primarily focused on emotional intimacy, with or without sexual intimacy. Poly relationships have a few distinctive characteristics, including the degree of sexual exclusivity, number of people involved, and level of emotional intimacy and commitment.

LEVELS OF SEXUAL EXCLUSIVITY

Sexual exclusivity, probably the single most important and distinguishing factor of monogamous relationships, is not expected in polyamorous relationships. Levels of sexual exclusivity, however, are a popular topic of conversation among polyamorous people, and it is the subject of intense negotiation.

Those in polyamorous relationships generally attempt to maintain sexually, and (ideally) emotionally, intimate relationships with no promise of sexual exclusivity. For ease of conversation, people in mainstream poly communities in the United States tend to use *polyamory* as an umbrella term to encompass the practices of polyamory, polyfidelity, and polysexuality. In this book I will use *polyamory* and *poly* interchangeably as the umbrella terms, and I will specify if I mean something else like *polyfidelity*.

Polyfidelity

Polyfidelity most closely resembles a closed group marriage because, while the people in it might not be married, they do expect the others in the relationship to be sexually exclusive with people inside the relationship group. It differs from polyamory in that *polyfideles* (the term for someone who is a polyfidelitist) generally expect the people in their group to be sexually exclusive, and polyamorists generally do not. The majority of polyfidelitous groups require that people who want to join their group get tested for sexually transmitted infections (STIs) prior to having sex of any kind with any group member, much less unprotected sex (which requires fluid bonding, see the definition later in this chapter). Members of polyfidelitous groups often see each other as family members, regardless of the degree (or lack) of sexual contact within their relationships. The larger the group is, the more likely it is to have members who do not have sex with each other.

Polyfidelitous groups sometimes experience cheating, when a member sneaks outside of the approved group to have sex with someone else who either has not been tested or approved or who might have been actively disapproved by other group members. While most polyamorists talk about avoiding making rules about how people should feel about each other, some polyfideles express a strong preference that all group members share equal feelings of affection or love for each other member of the group. Such equality seems much easier for smaller groups (especially triads) to maintain, and bigger groups inevitably develop some relationships that are more intense than others. The essential difference between polyamory and polyfidelity is that the polyfideles expect sexual exclusivity within their specific group and the polyamorists do not. Some polyamorists characterized those in polyfidelitous relationships as practicing "monogamy plus" and harboring a "closed-minded and grasping" approach to relationships. Some polyfideles, on the other hand, scorned polyamorists as "swinger wanna-bes" or "just screwing around." Each camp claimed to define the "real" form of polyamory and judged the other's practice as defective.

Polysexuality

Polysexuality is the practice of having sex with multiple people, either simultaneously (as a form of group sex) or in concurrent, dyadic (two-person) relationships. Depending on whom you talk to, polysexuality can cover a wide range, from dating many people casually or having lots of sex to using public sex environments or attending sex parties and orgies. Ryan, a white man in his late thirties, identified differences between his feelings of polysexuality and polyamory. With polysexuality, "there doesn't have to be any love to have good sex, it can be a carnal connection." He viewed the Judeo-Christian condemnation of multiple-partner relationships as a fundamental rejection of polysexuality. "The Bible is all about polyamory, what else do they mean by 'love your neighbors'? But they get real freaked out by polysexuality, [laughing] that's for sure."

Those who emphasized the distinction between polyamory and polysexuality often asserted that people could not participate in both, simultaneously. Someone who was polyamorous but not polysexual might develop a sexual relationship with one person and polyaffective relationships with others. In this scenario, polysexual persons have sex with many people, but they most likely love only one or no one at all. Others asserted that polyamory and polysexuality could coexist in the same person, and they have different expressions depending on the relationship.

Polyaffectivity

Many respondents described emotionally intimate, sexually platonic relationships with their partners' partners. Inspired by poly community tradition, I coined the term *polyaffective* to describe nonsexual relationships among people in polyamorous relationships. Adult polyaffective relationships with other adults appear as cospouses or quasi siblings, and with children as coparents, aunts/uncles, or quasi older siblings. Children's relationships with each appear as quasi sibling, cousin, friend, and rival.

Poly Geometry

Poly geometry refers to the number of people involved in the relationship and how they are related to each other. The number of people in the relationship can vary from one to many, and it includes *poly singles*, *open couples*, *vees*, *triads*, *quads*, *moresomes*, and *intimate networks*. As the number of people in the relationship gets larger, the relationships become less stable and less common.

Poly Singles

Poly singles are people with wide-ranging attitudes toward conducting relationships. *Free agents* prefer to abstain from, or have not yet found, primary partnerships. *Seekers* are actively dating and searching for the ideal polyamorous relationship. The people who are *poly-for-now* are usually experimenting with polyamorous relationship styles while they are young, unattached, or recently split up from a serious relationship. Poly-for-nows usually plan to "settle down" in a monogamous relationship eventually but are not yet ready or have not yet found the right person for a serious monogamous relationship. Second in number only to open couples—the most common form of relationship among mainstream poly communities—poly singles are also quite common because newcomers, and those between relationships, are often single.

Open Couples

The most common form of polyamorous relationship is the *open couple*. Most open couples in mainstream poly communities are composed of a woman and a man in a committed, long-term relationship, who often live together (some married, others unmarried) and who date other people in addition to their primary partner. The defining characteristic of an open couple is that they have (or are willing to have) sexual relationships with people outside the couple. Open couples take many forms, from those who date independently to those who only date as a pair, *poly/mono* couples, and *fly-throughs*.

Most open couples, such as Summer and Zack, date others individually. Summer and Zack, both white, college-educated IT professionals, were an open couple who had been together for over thirty years. During their three decades together their relationship had been through many transitions, and some other partners had come and gone, but Summer and Zack stayed together. While they did occasionally cohabitate, most significantly with Jarvis, one of Summer's partners, they usually lived alone together and dated other people. Initially Summer and Zack established a few ground rules that helped their relationship thrive. For instance, if one of them had a lover come over to spend the night, the live-in and visiting lovers would share the guestroom and the other primary would sleep in the main bedroom. Later they came to know each other so well that rules were no longer necessary because they had internalized the ways they figured out to care for the relationship.

Some open couples date exclusively as a couple. Jane, a white woman in her late forties, and her husband Sam, a man in his early sixties, both bisexual, were a polyamorous open couple. They always dated others together, and either one of them could use *veto power* when choosing lovers. If one person vetoed another lover, then neither one of them could have sex with that other person. Sam has never invoked the veto, but Jane "uses it liberally" when she does not like who Sam has chosen or to "conserve his energy." Jane recognized the imbalance in their use of the veto, but she felt it balanced the relationship in other ways, saying, "I am the brakes and he is the accelerator." Sexuality was central to life for Jane and Sam—both Tantra[4] practitioners and teachers: they had sex with each other at least twice daily as part of their spiritual practice and both wanted daily group sex as well. Their ideal was mutually dating two couples at the same time.

Because open couples are so prevalent in polyamorous communities, there are many discussions about how to best maintain a relationship in light of the pressures, emotional rigor, and relational complexity associated with polyamorous relationships. Numerous support group meetings focus on topics such as integrating another partner, soothing bruised feelings, and suggesting avenues to personal growth that will enable people to deal with jealousy. Polyamorous literature also includes extensive advice and suggestions about the best way to proceed as an open couple.

The *poly/mono* is a variety of the open couple that includes one polyamorous person and one monogamous person in a serious, long-term relationship, often a marriage. Usually both members of the relationship could have additional partners, but the monogamist usually does not want to (or is physically/medically unable to) have more partners but allows his or her partner/spouse to have multiple relationships.

One such poly/mono couple was Ian and Meredith, a white couple in their early forties, married for twenty-two years. Ian wanted multiple-partner relationships and, while Meredith was reluctant to take outside lovers herself, she said that she was "fine" with Ian seeking additional lovers. Ian said that Meredith "has had a few external liaisons, she would rather use her time and energy to sculpt. That is her real passion, but unfortunately not her day job." Ian "loves her [Meredith] dearly" and spent an average of four nights a week at home with her. He also spent two nights a week with Shawna, his girlfriend with whom he shared many common interests. In explaining his relationship, Ian said that both Meredith and Shawna's wife, Nancy, "love to see us together 'cause it makes us so happy."

Not all poly/mono relationships go so smoothly, however, as evidenced by Sheryl's predicament. Sheryl, a white woman in her late forties, met Jack, a white man in his mid-fifties, while they were contra dancing, and she "instantly fell in love." When Jack explained to Sheryl that he was polyamorous, she initially decided not to get involved with him because "I didn't think I could handle it." Sheryl resolved to see Jack only as a dance partner, but eventually she fell even more deeply in love with him and "just gave in" to an open-couple relationship. "There are really parts of it I enjoy: the honesty, self-knowledge, he treats me great!" Even so, Sheryl remained uncomfortable with Jack's polyamorous sexuality. "When I really think about it, I want him all to myself and it hurts me that he wants to be with other women." Jack was sympathetic and willing to discuss her pain at length, but he was unwilling to be monogamous with anyone. He told me, "She knew what she was getting into that first night. This is who I am."

Some poly/monos deal with the difficulty of blending two relationship styles by using a "don't ask, don't tell" (DADT) strategy. These are romantic relationships in which the monogamous partner allows the polyamorous partner additional relationships but does not want to hear any of the details or meet the other partners. Some people in DADT relationships encourage their partners to have sexual liaisons only while traveling, others allow any type of sexual relationship as long as safer-sex protocols are observed, and still others sanction only online relationships, as long as participants never meet in person.

The Campo family had an important poly/mono relationship that has been ongoing for many years. Campo family members include: Lexi, a mother of one with two family partners; Samuel, Lexi's husband; Blake, Lexi's cohabitational partner; Zina, Samuel and Lexi's adolescent daughter; and Dia and Brian, Lexi's parents. Samuel, Dia, and Brian lived with Zina on a farm about an hour outside a liberal town in the Pacific Northwestern portion of the United States where Lexi shared a home with Blake. Blake and Lexi routinely visited the farm, and Zina frequently came in to town to stay with her mother and Blake, though Brian, Dia, and Samuel did not come to town as often. All white and with varying degrees of education, the Campos were struggling to make ends meet and sustain two households, although the income Lexi was able to earn at the job she kept by living in town subsidized the farm significantly. Samuel was the swim coach and manager of a local pool, and Brian and Dia cared for foster children on their ranch, along with many animals.

The Campo family had evolved slowly into its current configuration. Samuel and Lexi had married when they were fairly young, and shortly afterward Samuel was seriously injured. Lexi explained how that changed their lives and impacted their practice of polyamory:

> At one point my husband, Samuel, for three or fourish years, I was monogamous with my husband or celibate when he got in a bad car accident and had a traumatic brain injury that changed his personality dramatically. I kind of consider myself to be in a cosmically arranged marriage. I was initially married to the person I chose as a spouse for about six months, but after his accident he had a marked change in personality and we have become emotionally close again, mutually supportive . . . while he did not request monogamy I felt like the chaos after the accident required that I pull my energy into the relationship . . . I was not seeing anyone else for a while and once I was interested in seeing other people he was capable of requesting me to not do that for a while. Samuel has never asked me not to do this or not to be this way. He has said that will hurt me or that will make me sad, but he has never made a proactive request for me to be something I wasn't. But he was so unhappy at the idea and he was so needy that it just kept being put off for a while. Every four or six months I would stay up all night crying and he said he would support me in my choices but then forget about it until the next time he saw me crying and that went on for about three years. At first he was very much an egocentric, self-centered child for that time after the accident. I came to a decision to delay getting those needs met right after the accident, but let him know that I would have to return to being who I really am at some point.

Years of communicating and reestablishing their relationship allowed Samuel and Lexi to negotiate a poly/mono relationship in which both of their needs were met. Lexi's willingness to delay her desire for poly relationships for over three years gave Samuel the time he needed to heal and learn to trust Lexi as he got to know her again. Their patience and communication has produced positive results, in that the whole family appears to be quite comfortable with their polyamorous arrangement.

When I asked him how he felt about being monogamous while his wife was polyamorous, Samuel at first gave me monosyllabic answers like "fine, great." Later in the interview I returned to that question and Samuel responded:

> Samuel: You are just not going to be happy until I have something bad to say about that, huh? (laughing) It really is fine, I am sincerely OK with this. If I wanted other partners I could have them, but I am just not interested. Sex is not that important to me, and if I want to have sex Lexi is always happy to be with me, so that need is met. The ranch is a lot of work, and I am the only full-time employee of the Parks and Rec in town, so that takes up a lot of time and attention. In the summer I hire people to work at the pool, but the rest of the year it's just me. And I really love coaching [the local swim team]. Zina takes a lot of my time, too, in a good way. It's all good, in fact.

> Elisabeth: Does it ever get to be a drag, living out here with Lexi's parents while she's in town with Blake?

> Samuel: No, I get along great with Dia and Brian. Brian and I take care of the ranch, and Dia [who had lost her legs to diabetes and used a wheelchair], and Zina. It all goes fairly smoothly, and I really don't have any complaints. I like living in the country and working with the kids and the animals, this suits me just fine.

Samuel stated firmly that he was comfortable in his poly/mono relationship, and in her own interview Zina echoed his sentiment.

> Elisabeth: How do you feel about your dad being monogamous while your mom is polyamorous?

> Zina: I don't think about it that much. I don't really see anything wrong with it, I dunno. It's just that, he could have other partners if he wanted to, but he just doesn't or whatever, so, I don't really know why. We don't usually talk about it, occasionally, but not usually.

Sometimes when I'm picking on him I will say about some girl or something "you have a crush on her don't you?" And he will be like "I do not," so it usually gets brushed off or whatever. I can tell it doesn't hurt his feelings, it's not a sore spot the way he reacts. It's no big deal. We joke about it. We could talk about it seriously if we wanted to, we just haven't had a need for it.

Lexi and Samuel's poly/mono relationship went remarkably smoothly, more so than most poly/mono relationships of which I was aware. Regarding poly/mono relationships, Blake commented:

I was part of a poly/mono relationship for eighteen years . . . and will never, ever do it again. There are several folks in the local poly scene who are also in poly/mono relationships, as is one of my sweeties. There seem to be two distinct and radically different kinds of poly/mono relationships. The first one in which a poly person is involved with a mono person, and that monogamous person really, really wishes the polyamorous person were monogamous too. This is the type I was in. My ex-wife was monogamous and wanted a monogamous relationship; she agreed to polyamory only reluctantly, and it was a constant source of stress and tension between us. Sadly, the people who got the worst of that tension were those who were luckless enough to be my partners. I've never seen this kind of relationship work out well. I've especially never seen it work out well for any third parties who happen along. There are a zillion ways for a person who's resentful about polyamory to make life miserable for a newcomer without ever quite being direct about it. The second kind of poly/mono relationship is one in which a polyamorous person is involved with a person who is "monogamous" in the sense that he doesn't want any additional partners himself, but is totally fine with the polyamorous person being poly. This is the relationship my partner is in right now with her husband. This kind of relationship can work very well.

In the Campo family's case, everyone involved agreed that the poly/mono configuration was working well for the family. This outcome was possible only because of the care and patience with which Samuel and Lexi had negotiated their agreement.

Another form of open couple is the *fly-through*—an established couple who become interested in trying polyamory, but their first experience with new partners ends with such disastrous consequences that they do not want to do polyamory any more. Most fly-throughs leave the polyamorous community upon ending their poly relationships. Chapter 4 includes discussion of issues related to open couples, such as couple privilege, veto power, and "unicorn hunting."

Vees

Vees are relationships among three people, with one member who is intimately connected with each of the two others. The relationship between the other two nonlovers can range from virtual strangers, who are aware of and cordial with each other, through good friends, to enemies. The association between the two nonlovers is not as close as it generally is in a triad, a more intimate polyamorous grouping with three members.

Triads

Polyamorous triads are generally made up of three adults who are all sexually involved, commonly understood as a *ménage-a-trio*. While occasionally a triad will begin as a threesome, more often triads form when a single person joins an open couple or a larger group loses a member(s). Tina, a thirty-six-year-old white urban planner, has been involved in two separate triads with married couples across a period of several years. The first triad attended social events together and spent time at home with the couple's two children. "It was like I was a member of the family with them, hanging out and folding the laundry and stuff. The sex was not all that important, and didn't happen a lot." The second couple was more focused on Tina as a "sexual accessory. Really, the only reason they wanted me around was for group sexual activities. That did not last for very long." Triads, like any relationship, vary tremendously depending on who is involved, where they live, what kind of resources they have, and how they organize their relationships. Tina's second couple were characteristic of *unicorn hunters*—a heterosexual man and bisexual or heteroflexible woman looking for a bisexual woman who will (the cliché implies) fit in to the couple's life at their convenience, bringing no additional partners of her own, disappear or pass as a friend when being openly poly might embarrass or inconvenience the couple, and hopefully wants to take care of the children and do the laundry.

In other instances, three people form a cooperative and loving family with sexual relationships between some members and platonic relationships between others. These *polyaffective triads* are more emotionally intimate than vees, but they are less sexually interactive than polyamorous triads. The Tree polyaffective triad was composed of Bjorn, Gene, Leah, and a son, Will. Leah had a sexual relationship with both men, and the men (each heterosexual) were platonic cohusbands. Polyaffective triads with two men and one woman were some of the most lasting poly relationships I found, and when they broke up the men often helped each other remain in contact with the children (more so than in other families when the men had been lovers).

Quads

Quads, as the name suggests, are groups of four adults most commonly formed when two couples join, although they can also develop when a triad adds a fourth or a moresome loses a member(s). Notoriously unstable, conventional poly wisdom that "2 + 2 = 3" or "a quad makes a great triad" implies that most quads will lose someone to poly-style divorce.

The formerly monogamous couples of Monique and Edward and Alicia and Ben, all white and in their late thirties or early forties, formed the Mayfield quad when Monique and Edward's two daughters, Josie and Kate, were three and five years old. Monique worked as an administrative assistant, Edward as a computer network designer, and Ben as a music producer. Alicia had previously been injured and was disabled enough that paid work was difficult, but she was able enough to care for Kate, Josie, and many of the household chores. Edward recalled that they had been advised that quads were unstable:

> The whole quad, right, had gotten advice for, well-respected people that were in quads, they generally break down into triads or pairs or whatever, they break down into and of course we were in love so that was just so much gobbledygook. Now, one thing that's interesting about the quad and which where we went to these meetings at least I was so proud to talk about this. You know, you've got to be careful because there are six relationships amongst four people with three

people you only have three maybe four depending on how you pattern it out but you have to be careful and make sure everybody's
communicating. Well, that's all well and good but we weren't. It is
very easy to say, oh yeah, you need to communicate, but communicating and *saying you need to communicate* [his emphasis] are two
entirely different things.

The Mayfields eventually broke up, with Monique and Ben forming a
lasting relationship, pained distance between Monique and Alicia, and
divorces for both legally married pairs.

In some quads all of the members have sexual relationships with
each other either in groups or pairs, but more commonly people have
sexual relationships with some and others are platonic. Morgan Majek
(a white mother of two and office manager) remembered a quad she
had been in when she was in her late twenties with her husband, Carl (a
white father of two and real estate developer/city planner), then in his
early thirties, and another married couple, Josh and Jessica, both white
and in their late thirties who had been married for twelve years. Both
heterosexual, Carl and Josh each had sexual relationships with Morgan
and Jessica but not each other. The women, sometimes singly and
sometimes as a pair, had sexual relationships with each man. They did
not, however, tend to have independent sex alone together as a couple.

After two years of good times and bad, they could no longer maintain the emotional stress, and that dissolved the quad. Morgan, however, remained involved with all members for "as long as I could take it, I
just hated to let it die!" Eventually, even Morgan gave up on her attempts to reunite the quad and stopped seeing both Josh and Jessica.
Her poly journey did not end there, though, and we will hear more
about all of these families later in the book.

Moresomes

Moresomes, groups with five or more adult members, are larger, more
fragile, and more complicated than the quads. Jana Founder's moresome, which started with an open couple and progressed from a polyaffective triad and into a moresome, exemplified the tendency of large
polyamorous relationships to change over time. Jana, a forty-seven-
year-old[5] white editor and mother of one, and Mike, a fifty-two-year-

old white writer, married when they were quite young. After several years of monogamy, they opened their relationship and met George, with whom each established a deep connection. The three lived as a polyaffective triad for thirteen years, with sexual relationships between Jana and both men and a platonic relationship between George and Mike. Jana and Mike divorced but continued to cohabitate, and they remained emotionally and sexually intimate. Jana reported, "We didn't want any of us more connected than the other, and with a marriage between me and Mike it seemed like our relationship was somehow more important than the one we had with George, and it wasn't really. So we got divorced, but nothing really changed."

Eventually Jana met Sam, a fifty-three-year-old white computer consultant. Sam and Jana maintained a long-distance relationship for several years until they decided they were serious enough to attempt cohabitation. In the meantime, Mike met Michelle, a white forty-six-year-old writer, and they established a similarly serious relationship. The five of them founded a family, with spousal relationships between Jana and Sam, George, and Mike, and also between Michelle and Mike. Michelle and Jana had a polyaffective relationship, as did Mike, George, and Sam. Jana and Sam had a child, and the moresome remained together through Zachariah's birth.

After a year of motherhood, Jana felt raising Zachariah while maintaining such a complex web of relationships was taking a toll on her, so she, Sam, and Zachariah moved out of the home they had shared with the entire moresome. Michelle and Mike moved a few blocks away and maintained close contact with the rest of the family. George lived with Sam and Jana for six months of every year, spending the other six months with a lover in Hawaii. Zachariah saw Michelle, George, and Mike regularly, and he continued to think of them as his family. Although the moresome changed over time, the core family connection remained.

Intimate Network

One step larger than a moresome, an *intimate network* is a group of closely connected people who do not generally cohabitate as a unit (though some segments might cohabitate) and are sexually intimate with various group members. Some intimate networks consider themselves families, though most do not. Intimate networks often have entrance procedures that include disclosure of, and testing for, sexually transmitted infections (STIs). These procedures include a discussion of appropriate precautions against transmission, as well as the specific norms and boundaries that structure member's expanded relationships.

Thaddeus, a thirty-five-year-old white musician, remembered how an intimate network of twenty men[6] introduced him to the polyamorous community:

> About twenty men in a relationship and I was *astounded* and it was a good thing that this was a closed relationship because if it'd been open I would have tried to dive in and, at seventeen [years old], would have ended up being something of a bull in a china shop. I'm sure. It was beautiful to see. They were all over thirty-five and I was seventeen and obviously it just would not have functioned probably to their expectations. I think it would have been beyond mine. They had that number because a lot of them traveled and didn't want to play around on the side because it's [the AIDS epidemic] scary. And the reason why I think it would have been a bull in a china shop situation is that I wasn't stable. I had been coming from a rather difficult childhood. I would have invested an awful lot of [pause] an awful lot of energy in just trying to be whatever they would have needed me to be. And with twenty of them, all of them are highly attractive men I just feel like I would have torn a swath and caused problems and that's been something I've worked most of my life not to do.

While Thaddeus admired this network of men, there was an undertone of caution in his tale. That a visiting adolescent could "tear a swath" underlines his belief that the expanded relationship between the men are fragile, a delicately balanced unit that could inadvertently be destroyed.

Most large networks maintain brief (usually several months to several years) stability, and then membership changes. I interacted briefly with a member of another intimate network of twenty gay men in the San Francisco Bay area that owned a large house together. Two members had recently moved out to cohabit monogamously. The remaining men began searching for two new members. The member in attendance at the party quipped, "If you think it is hard to date others as a couple, just think about how hard it is for us to date a couple as eighteen!" He laughed, but his underlying message was clear: maintaining such a large and complex intimate network was a challenging and intricate task.

LEVEL OF INTIMACY AND COMMITMENT

In addition to the level of sexual exclusivity and numbers of people involved, polyamorists frequently categorized their relationships by their levels of intimacy, commitment, and duration.

Primary, Secondary, and Tertiary

Community members often use the terms *primary*, *secondary*, and (less often) *tertiary* to describe their varied levels of connection. Primary partners—sometimes corresponding to the larger cultural conception of a spouse—usually have long-term relationships, joint finances, cohabit, mutually make major life decisions, and some have children. Secondary partners share an emotional connection but tend to keep their lives more separate than primary partners. Secondaries often discuss major life decisions, but they do not usually make those decisions jointly. They typically have separate finances and residences, and some have less intense emotional connections than do primary partners. Tertiary relationships are usually allotted less time and energy than primary and secondary relationships. Although possibly the first phase of a deeper relationship or an enduring long-distance relationship, more often relationships with tertiary partners are less emotionally intimate and can resemble swinging.

These definitions, like so much in the polyamorous subculture, are subject to varied interpretations by polyamorists. Tina described a group discussion in which her partner, Edward Mayfield, changed his mind about her classification:

> And he was saying that he feels that since he's married that Monica [his wife] should be primary and I should be secondary. I was like, okay, whatever. As much as I was like, I don't know how that's going to work out so well. But it has been working out just fine. And secondary is secondary. You feel like, well, how is this secondary? In

what ways is it secondary? So we were having this discussion at a group over at a potluck sometime about how do you define your primaries and your secondaries. And one person was saying I define it by, well, I don't have any secondaries, everybody is a primary. And she was saying—and somebody else was saying well I define it by the amount of time I spend with that person or however many primaries they have. I become a secondary. So after that conversation, Edward turned to me and said well, I guess we must be primaries because we spend a lot of time together.

Similarly, Morgan described the fluidity that defined what she and the other members of her quad thought of as primary or secondary:

Carl is primary in that we're living together, he supports us, and I feel like, yeah, it's still primary. If we were to all live together, it would be equal I'd have two primaries. Josh feels, I think, I don't know how you can have another primary and not be living together. Because Josh considers me equal with Jessica, but they're still primary. It's because they're living together . . . It's different when you're actually living with someone. You don't, you answer to them differently. Just more, you know, it's more of a primary relationship.

Polys often disagree about specific definitions of primary, secondary, and tertiary; some refuse the distinctions altogether, preferring what they cast as "less hierarchical" and "more compassionate" terminology.

Nesting/Non-Nesting

Polyamorous people regularly debate the categorization of relationships. Some view the primary/secondary/tertiary terminology as hierarchical and contrary to their desire for more compassionate forms of relationship. These people prefer *nesting* and *non-nesting* to differentiate between partners who live together and others who maintain intimate emotional lives but keep their residences, finances, and decisions separate. Thinking back on her poly triad, Melody Lupine, a thirty-six-year-old white magazine editor and mother of three, asserted that she did not feel that any of her lovers were primary to her, not only because she felt uncomfortable placing some beneath the others, but also:

My number one relationship is with myself. And one thing I've learned is polyamory helps me, especially as a woman, to keep my autonomy so that I don't lose myself, whether it be within a relationship, like a man or a woman or my children. It helps me to define what I want and set my boundaries and take relationships at what I need.

Joya Starr, a mother of one and a costume designer, feels more comfortable focusing on a certain group synergy than on the type of relationship:

Very rarely do I "primary partner." It's not my natural bent. I like ones, threes, and fives the best. I like myself a lot. I have been in some long-term triads where the energy for that really flows very well and I think has a stability that I haven't found in other numbers. But I would say my favorite is five because I really love boys together a lot and I don't get that in my triads.

Joya values the quality of interaction between people, and she feels that categories such as primary or non-nesting did not reflect her experience. She largely rejects primary partnerships:

I haven't found in myself that ability to care for one partner more than my other partners. I've had places where I feel like I'm more expressed with one than the other, but I mean, there were times where it would be like, OK, is it the one that I've been involved with for a decade, is it the one that I had a child with, is it the one that makes my body sing, is it the one who I can talk to and explore the place when you are in conversation about what you don't already know, when you get into that kind of magic kind of talking. And I couldn't for the life of me say that one of those people were more primary to me than the other, like I needed all of that and more, and I felt whole not with one more than the other.

Some polys who reject hierarchical distinctions between lovers discard the notion of primaries relating altogether. For them, relating to lovers around a specific quality makes the differences among primary/secondary and nesting/non-nesting insignificant. These polys often point out that both categorizations relied upon the same distinction: the degree of practical interdependence was the truly important quality, rather than emotional depth.

USEFUL TERMS

Because polyamory is a relatively recent and unusual relationship innovation, conventional English provides few (if any) words to describe openly conducted, nonmonogamous relationships. Polyamorists have thus been forced to create their own words to reflect and describe their own experiences, several of which appear below.

- *Compersion* (termed *frubbly* in the United Kingdom) is the joy at seeing one's partner(s) happily in love with others. It is not precisely the opposite of jealousy, but close.
- *Fluid bonding* is when people decide that they are willing to exchange bodily fluids during sexual encounters. Poly community norms dictate that, unless otherwise explicitly negotiated, everyone is assumed to be having safer sex in which no fluids will be transferred.
- A *metamour* or an OSO (Other's Significant Other) is the partner of a partner (a girlfriend's boyfriend), people who do not share a sexual connection with each other but do have a partner in common. Metamours and OSOs are aware of each other and are usually friends or acquaintances, but they occasionally become enemies or rivals.
- *New Relationship Energy* or *NRE* is a term coined by Zhahai Stewart[7] to describe the overwhelming rush of love, characteristic of the beginnings of relationships when everything is exciting, new, and exhilarating.
- *Polyaffectivity* is the term I have coined for emotionally intimate poly relationships that are nonsexual. People in poly relationships who see each other as family members but are not sexually connected (for instance, spice [see below] who share a lover in common but are not lovers themselves) have polyaffective relationships.
- The *polyamorous possibility* is what I call the mind-set that acknowledges the potential to love multiple people at the same

time, or the awareness of polyamory as a relationship option. Once it has occurred to someone that openly conducted, multiple-partner relationships are possible and can be managed in an ethical manner, they can never unthink that idea. They have become aware of the polyamorous possibility and, regardless of whether they consider polyamory themselves or simply reject it out of hand, they can never again be unaware of consensual nonmonogamy as an option.

- *Spice* are multiple spouses.
- *Swolly* is a term coined by Ken Haslam[8] to describe the intersection between swinging and polyamory, where the two different styles of nonmonogamy overlap and become difficult to distinguish.
- The *unicorn* is an unattached bisexual woman who wants to date (or simply have a quick ménage a trios) an existing female/male couple. She is so rare as to be virtually mythical. In her most exaggerated form, she is a young, single woman, eager to move to the couple's dilapidated farm in rural North Dakota to care for their children, work on their farm, clean their house, be their sex toy, and disappear whenever it would be inconvenient to explain her presence to the couples' family or friends.

COMMON GUIDELINES THAT STRUCTURE POLYAMOROUS RELATIONSHIPS

1. *There are no rules* that everyone has to follow. Each relationship makes their own guidelines, which tend to share a few common themes. Other than that, polyamorists have what one poly person called "designer relationships" in that each group can make their individual relationship whatever they wish it to be.
2. *Tell the truth.* It is impossible to feel safe without trust, and trust flourishes with honest communication.
3. *Communicate, communicate, communicate.* This helps to clarify expectations, manage complexity, and develop intimacy.
4. *If he gets more lovers then so does she* (and vice versa). While there are poly/mono couples in which one partner is polyamorous and the other is monogamous, most commonly the monogamous

people have the option to have other lovers and simply do not avail themselves of it.

5. *Make and follow safer sex agreements*, or negotiated contracts among lovers stipulating what kinds of sex they can have with other people and how exactly they will protect against sexually transmitted infections. Popular elements include requiring extensive use of prophylactics (condoms, gloves, and dental dams), testing for sexually transmitted infections, and immediate disclosure of any infections.

6. *Take responsibility for self-growth*, even if it is uncomfortable. Jealousy and insecurity are serious issues for many people in poly relationships, and the desire to exert veto power the moment these feelings become unmanageable can be overwhelming.

7. *Allow for change.* Not only do poly relationships often work out differently than people had anticipated that they might, but they also tend to change over time. If the people in them are not willing to change with them, things fall apart fairly rapidly.

8. And most important of all: *Treat people kindly and live an ethical life.* Or as the popular poly saying goes, "Don't be a dick." This guideline extends to everyone, not just lovers. In general, be willing to give others the benefit of the doubt, assume they are trying their hardest, treat them gently, and let ethical considerations guide behaviors.

2

WHO DOES POLYAMORY, AND WHY?

Most people in mainstream polyamorous communities in the United States and those who volunteer to participate in research on poly relationships—my own research and others'[1] —are white, middle or upper-middle class, highly educated, and employed in professional fields such as information technology, counseling, or education. The people in my study shared some personality traits that were also common in poly communities, such as being liberal, intellectual, open-minded, geeky, and devoted to social justice. They are aging hippies, young professionals, science fiction enthusiasts obsessed with steampunk, and families with children. Like the general population, the vast majority of polys are *cis-gendered*, meaning that they identify with the body and gender in which they were born. Most are not *transgendered* (people whose external sex or gender does not match their internal experiences of themselves) or *intersexed* (people with a blend of chromosomes or ambiguous genitalia that means they are a mix of both male and female, used to be called hermaphrodite).

WHO DOES POLYAMORY? WHO IS POLYAMOROUS?

While these two questions appear to be synonymous, they are actually quite different for polyamorists. Much like some monogamous people grit their teeth and force themselves to ignore or repress attractions for others (doing monogamy) and other monogamous people are simply and profoundly uninterested in other possible romantic partners when they are in a relationship (monogamy by orientation), polyamorists can approach the relationship style in a variety of ways, or combine several approaches at once. Some people *do* polyamory, meaning they see it as an option, a lifestyle, or even a form of sacred sexuality practice they may choose depending on the circumstances in their lives and relationships. This group envisioned polyamory as a spiritual path based on practices of honesty, self-knowledge, and sacred sex, or a practice that augmented other forms of spirituality such as Paganism, Tantra, Taoism, or Quodoshka.[2] Rosie, the leader of a sacred sexuality group popular among a small group of polyamorists, pointed out:

> The vast majority of polys seek a deeper connection on all levels. They are seekers of knowledge, and sacred sex takes sex beyond, "OK, let's jump in the sack and get laid"—it takes sex to a much deeper connection. . . . Poly people are explorers, they are more open-minded and they seek alternatives to enhance their lives and have more real relationships. Sacred sex does that for them.

These polys craved and created in practice an integration between the Divine and the physical body that acted as a form of spirituality. People who practiced a form of sacred sexuality often linked a personal connection with the Divine to their increasingly intimate emotional and sexual connection with others.

Others saw polyamory as a lifestyle (or a "lovestyle" in poly lingo), a choice that gave polys much greater relationship flexibility than monogamists usually allowed themselves (at least openly). Polyamorists with this belief tended to emphasize freedom as central to their relationships and identities. Emmanuella Ruiz—a university professor and mother of three in her mid-forties—stated:

> It's about what I've been saying, a broader base of community can be built and shared and that if I choose to share my body with people within that constellation, that's my choice. And if I don't want to, that's my choice too.

Members of this group often avoided activism and other activities that might draw public attention (and attendant discrimination) to polyamory. Many thought it best to "pass" and had chosen to "blend in" and use their misattributed access to "monogamous privilege" to their own advantage.

For others, polyamory is a *belief or worldview* based on abundance, multiplicity, and freedom. In some cases, people who are new to the idea of polyamory practice it as a belief before finding a partner with whom they can practice it in action (poly in theory). In other cases, some community leaders view polyamory as a movement intent upon securing equal rights and educating monogamous people regarding polyamorists and the issues they confronted. Those who viewed themselves as activists on behalf of the movement quipped that they were "polyactive." They made a variety of public appearances on radio and television broadcasts, granted newspaper interviews, spoke to public groups, wrote books, hosted conferences and workshops, and edited magazines.

A New York group called Polyamorous NYC was perhaps one of the most publicly visible organizations, having hosted an annual Poly Pride Day at Great Hill in Central Park annually since 2001. Polyamorous NYC hoped to promote awareness and acceptance of polyamory with the pride day, as well as bring community members together in a festival atmosphere. Small by public march standards, there were about one hundred attendees at the first gathering in 2001 and 150 the next year. Some attendees traveled from as far away as Seattle and Kentucky.[3] Finally, some people *are* polyamorous, meaning it functions as an essential or innate sexual or relationship orientation in their lives.

Members of this latter group who experience polyamory as a sexual or relational orientation often report knowing they wanted multiple partners even as children and feeling profoundly uncomfortable in the monogamous relationships they did attempt. Joya Starr, a costume designer and mother of one, reported that, when she had previously been in monogamous relationships, she

> felt suffocated, as if my skin were crawling and I couldn't breathe. And I always ended up cheating and felt terrible about it. I never meant to hurt anyone but could not wrap my head around how to be exclusive with just one person when there were so many people in the world. By the end of high school I was not making monogamous agreements with anyone anymore, and haven't for the last 20 years now.

Lexi Campo, a white customer service professional and mother of one, also felt that she was polyamorous by orientation: "I have always been poly. When I was four years old I told my caretaker that I would have a wife and we would share three or four husbands. I have always had a multiple-adult ideal in my head." When I asked if she had ever been monogamous, Lexi replied:

> Not really. I was both celibate and monogamous in behavior for sections of our marriage, after my husband, Samuel, had a bad accident that severely injured his brain. For about three or four years I was physically monogamous, though I maintained cyber-relationships with people who were emotionally supportive of me, and that included some cybersex. Samuel knew all about it and was OK with it . . . I have a very high libido and am very motivated by touch and cuddling. At a very basic level I want more than one partner in my life and if I don't have that I don't do as well. More importantly, I like to be surrounded by people and creating a schedule and having dinner as a group, laughing and noisy. On a fundamental level I like being surrounded by that kind of collective energy . . . communal living is very important to me.

Lexi wondered if there was a biological component to her polyamorous orientation, stating that:

> Gayness and bisexuality are common on both sides of my natal families, as is multiple partners relating with mistresses and wives or multiple partners for many important relatives all the way back to 1604 when two brothers both lived with a woman for 40 years, and while it is not clear who slept with whom, they lived as a three-person unit.

Lexi's parents Brian and Dia reported a long-term triadic relationship in their own past, supporting Lexi's assertion that "poly might run in my genes." Whether or not there was a genetic component to desire for multiple partners, the fact that Lexi believed that there was reinforced her image of herself as innately polyamorous.

COMMUNITY CHARACTERISTICS

Age

Most of the people in the study were in their early thirties to mid-sixties, though there are certainly older and younger segments of the polyamorous population. This age distribution makes sense for at least three reasons. First, my focus has been on families with children, and most middle-class families with kids in the United States today have parents that are in their thirties and forties. Second, the poly pioneers of the 1960s and 1970s (what I call the second wave of polyamory) are still around, and some of them are eager to talk to researchers because they are pleased to see polyamory finally getting serious attention. Third, because poly relationships are outside the norm and have to be consciously negotiated, it often takes people a while to try them. Many people follow social conventions early in life out of ingrained training, lack of power to make other choices, or sheer habit. Discomfort with social norms or desire for alternatives may take years to germinate and grow in to taking action toward stepping outside of accepted norms and values. Because polyamory challenges one of the most cherished contemporary social norms—monogamy—it can be intimidating to broach and is often not the first step in a journey beyond conventional social bounds.

The *polygeezers*, organized by Ken Haslam,[4] who coined the term, are a growing group of older polys, some of whom have been having multiple-partner relationships for many years and others of whom embark upon poly relations once their adult children are distracted with their own lives or after losing a spouse to death or divorce. As the baby boomers age and polyamory continues to grow in popularity, I predict that this segment of the poly population will expand dramatically. Retirement communities and nursing homes have already begun dealing with issues generated by residents in poly (as well as same-sex) relationships.[5]

People in their twenties are certainly practicing polyamory, and some consciously identify it as such, but they have not been as interested in participating in my research and tend not to have children, so they were not my focus. As I will explain later with sexual orientation, if a group already has a built-in mechanism to deal with nonmonogamy, then they are less likely to emerge as a significant subpopulation in poly communities. The college hook-up culture is so common among white, middle-class youth that it can make a polyamorous identity, with its tinge of families with kids and aging hippies, less compelling for many people in their twenties.

Gender

One of the most distinguishing characteristics of polyamory is that it allows women multiple partners. Across time, most multiple-partner relationship styles have allowed men multiple wives (polygyny) but only rarely do women "get" multiple husbands (polyandry). When a woman is married to multiple men, they tend to be brothers or some other form of a preestablished social group, and the woman is often required to perform wifely tasks (cooking, cleaning, sex, childrearing) for them all.[6] Far more frequently, polygamy is organized as polygyny, which is also more common than monogamy across history and various cultures.

This emphasis on gender equality has significant implications for poly relationships. Although there are certainly important poly men in communities and as researchers, women have historically dominated leadership positions in both poly communities and in academic circles that study these groups. While equality is a complex and elusive ideal that can be difficult to achieve or sustain, in practice poly women often do have equal—and in some instances greater—power than either monogamous women or poly men. Much of this is class based: poly women tend to be highly educated and frequently able to support themselves financially, which gives them the autonomy to contemplate the end of the relationship without the dread of possibly ending up living in their cars with their children. As is also true for economically self-sufficient women in monogamous relationships, the ability to leave means that poly women are much less likely to tolerate objectionable relationship conditions. Being able to set firm boundaries and make relationship requirements is both a source and an expression of power that is denied women in most traditional or patriarchal marriages, and even more so in most contemporary polygynous marriages that are often based in religious systems that require women to submit to male dominance.

In addition to social class, poly women have the poly-specific advantage of being more highly sought-after partners. Whether a result of the enduring sexual double standard that allows men far greater sexual latitude than women or a biological propensity that compels them to spread their seed, men seem more willing to have multiple partners. While women outnumber men in a few poly communities, in general there are fewer women available to spark new relationships. This comparative rarity can provide poly women with a numerical and social advantage because they have more options than their male counterparts.

Bisexuality plays a significant role in poly women's social advantage, as well. The ability to be attracted to both genders not only allows the women to consider a far wider range of potential partners but also gives bisexual women the added social cache of being the "hot bi babe" (or HBB)[7] that so many female-male couples want to add to their existing relationships. This social dynamic of a couple—usually a heterosexual man and a woman who is bisexual, bicurious, or heteroflexible—looking for a bisexual woman is so common in poly circles that it is cliché. These eligible bisexual women are so rare that polys (and swingers) call them "unicorns," and the couples who want to hook-up and/or establish relationships with them are labeled "unicorn hunters." The cliché holds that (most often at the male's behest) unicorn hunters will approach a poly community either in person or online with a list of what they seek in a female partner. Usually this includes someone who is bisexual, unattached (meaning not bringing in her own partners as well), wants to help raise the children, clean the house, have sex with the couple, and disappear when it would be inconvenient to explain her presence. Poly community responses to these gaffes vary from encouraging the unicorn hunters to think about why the women would want them and what they have to offer in addition to what they want from her, to "flaming" in which the unicorn hunters are shamed and badgered until they leave (this happens primarily online). Chapter 4 addresses these issues in greater detail.

The men who are drawn to poly relationships tend to be interested in social justice and egalitarian relationships. Because polyamory contrasts sharply with other multiple-partner relationship styles in which men are allowed multiple women but are not required to share their female partners with other men, the men who select polyamory as an alternative to monogamy or polygyny must be willing to step outside of an ownership model. Not that all poly men are paragons of equality or that the ideal always lives in reality, but to be willing to consider sharing a woman with another man requires a flexible personality and openness to equality that goes against conventional masculinity that demands that "real" men have unquestioned, exclusive access to "their" women.[8] The poly men I interviewed often did not insist on sexual ownership of women, tended to be liberal, open-minded, and invested in social and gender justice (something I call *polyhegemonic masculinity*).[9]

Sexual Orientation

While there is considerable variation, in my research and in mainstream poly communities there are mostly heterosexual men and bisexual women, with a significant minority of heterosexual women and a smaller minority of bisexual men.[10] The dominance of heterosexuality among men mirrors larger society in which most people identify as heterosexual. Bisexual men's comparatively lower status also mirrors both monogamous and swinging cultures in which women's bisexuality is highly valued as entertaining to men who, as Marlie, a thirty-seven-year-old white woman, put it, "get to watch while women warm each other up and then come in and finish them off with the big penis-inator." In sharp contrast, male bisexuality is cast as threatening to heterosexual masculinity and unappealing to women.

Another reason for the emphasis on heterosexuality and bisexuality is that both of these sexual orientations have traditionally been less developed as identities and thus do not already have an existing social niche. As the social norm, heterosexuality is so dominant that it remains unquestioned and is rarely taken as a primary identity. Much like whiteness masquerades as a nonrace, heterosexuality usually blends in to the social background unless something specifically emphasizes it. Bisexuality is often invisible, mistaken as homo or heterosexuality, and historically marginalized from or absorbed by gay and lesbian communities. Heterosexual and bisexual people who seek community based on shared sexual or relationship proclivity are required to build it for themselves, and they do so following a similar route blazed by gays and lesbians (who in turn patterned their political movement on the civil rights movement).

There are few exclusively same-sex relationships among polyamorous men, primarily because, as a friend once told me, "Gay men invented open relationships, we don't need another label to do what we are already doing." Lesbians also have nonmonogamous norms and groups already within their own communities, and they may be reluctant to join poly gatherings because of the potential to encounter unwanted male attention. I discuss reasons for the relative lack of people in exclusively same-sex relationships in greater detail in chapter 3.

Race and Class

Having unconventional relationships can be dangerous: The stigma associated with nonmonogamy means that being exposed as a polyamorist can result not only in strained relationships with families of origin and friends but also job loss, eviction from housing, and losing custody of children. For white, middle-class people, race and class privileges shield them from some of the potential impacts of nonconformity and provide resources to deal with disadvantages or discrimination. People already laboring under the disadvantages of poverty and racism—externally fixed social realities that are difficult or impossible to change—are less likely to be willing or able to take on additional stigma voluntarily. Similarly, those who receive public assistance are under far more surveillance than are those who do not. Living in public housing or receiving food stamps means disclosing roommates, partners, and relationships to authorities, and living with multiple partners (even secretly) can result in the denial of housing or monetary benefits.

People with enough money to own their homes, attain the kind of education that makes them indispensible at work or able to be self-employed, and sufficient funds to hire good lawyers in case their mother-in-law seeks custody of their children have the latitude to take the risks associated with voluntary nonconformity. White people can do whatever they want without worrying about being seen as examples of their entire race, whereas, stereotypically, people of color are already labeled as dangerously hypersexual and run the risk of being used as proof of how "those people" have loose morals or bad values.[11]

I began this research in Colorado, a state that is predominantly white, and my initial sample was composed largely of white people with a few people of color. In an attempt to get a more diverse sample, I traveled to the California Bay Area to collect data in one of the most diverse areas of the nation with one of the largest known poly communities. In defiance of my best efforts, even in the Bay Area I found mostly white, middle-class poly people, and it has been difficult for me to find respondents of color to interview. While this seems as if it is beginning to shift now, there just weren't that many people of color in mainstream polyamorous communities when I started this research, and those people of color who are involved might be less willing to participate in research than their white counterparts who volunteered in droves.

The people of color who did participate in interviews gave several reasons why there might be so few people of color in mainstream poly communities. In addition to the dangers of surveillance and risks of job or housing loss, people of color risk rejection from their ethnic or racial communities and the possibility that white people in poly communities will stereotype or objectify them. Yansa, a twenty-nine-year-old kink- and poly-identified African American[12] health care provider, said she was extremely uncomfortable when she attended a house party in the San Francisco Bay Area in which most attendees were playing in a backyard swimming pool.

> I was not sure if they wanted me there. Like I felt like maybe I had walked in on somebody else's thing and I wasn't invited. . . . [there were] seventy-five, eighty naked people in this huge pool and I walked in and everybody just turned and looked . . . and I realized I am the only black person here. I was the only person in a swimming suit so that could have been another issue, too, like maybe she's lost her way, what is she doing here?

Not only the sole black person at the party, as the only person in a swimsuit Yansa felt as if she stood out even more. Though organizers called the event "clothing optional," meaning that people could wear clothes or not depending on their personal tastes, the community norm was that people were naked while in the swimming pool and wore whatever they wanted (nudity to full dress) on the pool deck.

While Yansa became progressively more comfortable socializing in her local poly community, she became increasingly nervous about the possible backlash from other people if they found out she was polyamorous. At one point she was the only black employee in her section of a large financial institution, and she was certain that if they found out she was poly they would fire her, because her employers were

> executives who went to Wharton and Harvard and were Republicans and assholes . . . very, very closed minded. And I got the impression that they were already not comfortable with me being a person of color. To throw in the other stuff that I did may confirm their stereotypes about black people or they may have just thought she's the weirdest shit on the planet, I don't trust her . . . We don't want her on this job anymore, someone may find her out.

Because she was unique in her environment and already faced the racism that permeates contemporary society in the United States, Yansa felt that she had to carefully guard her secret poly identity lest its disclosure confirm stereotypes her employers most likely held. In this instance, racism acted as a significant deterrent to Yansa's ability to be comfortably out as a poly person.

Not only did Yansa experience forces in conventional society repelling her from identifying as a polyamorist but also she reported discussions with other African Americans who were judgmental of or could not understand her involvement in poly relationships.

> I've heard from black folks that they think it's a nasty white person thing to do. And they throw out the whole scenario of slavery you know they raped us and they took our women and impregnated them and . . . that any respectable, educated, cultured black person in their right mind wouldn't even think about doing something so disgusting.

Not only are poly relationships a "nasty white person thing" and "disgusting" for these "black folks," they are also rife with the potential for sexual stereotype and exploitation.

> I've had black people in the community tell me that they don't want to feel like the token black . . . the novelty like the fat girl or the Asian girl. I don't want to feel like people are attracted to me and wanting to play with me or date me because they're trying to figure

out something. Like I'm some anthropological experiment or something.

Yansa reported that the black people she knew rejected poly subcultures as white, foreign, and potentially corrupt social environments in
which the white majority might see the black people in attendance as
merely sex toys rather than multifaceted potential partners.

Like Yansa, Victor, a poly-identified thirty-six-year-old African
American therapist, artist, and college instructor, thought the black
people he knew would not approve of polyamory. "I can imagine being
in a room of black people and them going that sounds like crazy white
folks, that's some crazy shit." Victor felt more comfortable in his local
poly community than Yansa felt in hers, and even though it was "mono-
chromatic," Victor was not sure if that resulted from "issues of either
privilege or even cultural interest." The fact that nearly all of his poly
friends were white did not particularly bother him, partially because he
grew up around white people and felt he was "acclimated" to them.
Victor also thought that his poly friends seemed less racist than other
people he knew in conventional society. "People who are interested in
really relating with people and good whole truth telling are going to
tend to be less racist . . . I've actually felt a lot of acceptance."

Not only did the apparent lower levels of racism make Victor feel at
home in his local poly community, he also said that his education and
work background allowed him to experiment with relationships in a way
that other people with less privilege might not find accessible.

> It's sort of privilege related . . . if you're not worrying about certain
> things, then you have the privilege or the space to explore alterna-
> tives. . . . the freedom to explore polyamory sort of comes from a
> freedom either financially or just psychologically not having to
> [struggle to] survive in other ways.

Victor saw polyamorous relationships as less accessible to people who
were forced by racism and poverty to struggle to survive, and he acknowledged that his class and education privileges allowed him to live
more comfortably in his poly community.

This is not to say that African Americans are not having multiple-
partner relationships: Black people in the United States do have nonmonogamous relationships, but they might be less likely to label them

as polyamorous than their white counterparts. Victor thought it was unlikely that mainstream African Americans would embrace an organized poly identity, even though there were "communities of color where there are multipartner relationships going on. I don't know whether they would call it poly or not. Probably not. . . . I think that populations tend to self select."

Mikayla, a twenty-eight-year-old African American woman who worked as an educational consultant and performing artist and identified as bisexual, engaged in what she (in retrospect) saw as poly relationships, though they had not defined them so at the time.

> Deep down I think a lot of African American men are poly and just not open about it. They have the characteristics—do things that poly people do without saying it or admitting it so people call it cheating. I meet so many young men here in Georgia with multiple kids with multiple women, and that is a freakin' poly relationship to me. They can say cheater, when they see many women at the same time, but it sounds like to me deep down you are poly. I guess when you move from cheating to being open is when it can actually be defined as poly.

Mikayla reported that the black people she knew not only routinely engaged in de facto poly relationships but also that they were inflected with an entrenched sexual double standard that allowed men far more latitude than women.

> The act of poly versus the philosophy of poly—no, philosophically they are cheating. But the act—being in multiple homes, living with multiple women or in on and off relationships that sounds to me like poly . . . There is a silence in the African American community so certain things are not communicated but it is probably obvious . . . This is taboo, even though I am doing it. It is fine to do it as long as you don't talk about it . . . There remains a double standard there. I think [my boyfriend] Marlon knows that it happens—the women he is involved with having relationships with other men—but I know there is a double standard. He used to speak frequently about not trusting hoes (women in general and women he was involved with).

There is no question that some people—not only African Americans but also every other race or ethnicity—engage in nonmonogamous relationships but do not identify as polyamorous.

Similarly, there are undoubtedly people who identify as polyamorous but do not attend meetings or join groups. Again, it could be that those who feel marginalized or different from the more "visible" members of poly communities will remain outside the very organizations that purportedly represent their ilk. It is also possible that people of color involved in unconventional sexual practices are just as active but more clandestine and maintain their own, more exclusive, list-serves, events, and private sexual venues. Precisely how these more underground sexual networks might differ from the more visible sexual subcultures requires additional research.[13]

Who Is Missing?

For the reasons I explore above, the most obvious group missing from mainstream poly communities is people of color, although recent shifts in crowd composition at poly events seem to indicate a trend toward greater racial and ethnic diversity among poly communities in the California Bay Area and the Southeastern United States. If poly communities continue to follow in the wake of LGBTQ communities, they will become increasingly racially and ethnically diverse. Still in short supply, working-class people and those in exclusively same-sex relationships remain scarce in mainstream poly communities. Working class or poor people may not have the time or the finances to pursue multiple-partner relationships because maintaining multiple relationships is so time-consuming that it can interfere with holding multiple jobs, something that many working-class and poor people must do to cope with rising prices and stagnant low wages. Much of the poly community organizing and communicating happens online, and to access the poly sites it is almost crucial to have private high-speed Internet. Libraries often censor sexually explicit materials, and they may define any discussion of sexuality—of which there is plenty on poly websites—as sexually explicit and thus restrict access to these sites on public access computers.

Another group of people who do not appear in these data are conservatives in multiple-partner relationships. Poly communities in the United States have a decidedly liberal tone, and those who are both conservative and poly do not have much social space to espouse their ideals publicly. Occasionally Christian polyamorists will approach online communities and are routinely badgered or shunned as illegitimate polyamorists because (for the most part) the husbands are the only ones allowed multiple wives but the wives are required to be monogamous with the husband. This type of relationship fits better with a polygynous model than a polyamorous one, but some of these husbands identify as polyamorous and approach online groups looking for additional wives—with generally poor results. Other research indicates that swingers are more politically conservative than polyamorous people, and religious polygnists also tend to be far more traditional and patriarchal than do poly folks.[14] Other nonmonogamists who openly maintain multiple-partner relationships but do not identify as polyamorous do not appear in this research. I would have been interested in talking to them, but it was challenging enough to focus on poly-identified people that expanding the study to include other versions of nonmonogamy was beyond the scope of the project.

Another group that is almost completely absent is composed of those people who used to be polyamorous but are no longer. Researchers who conduct studies while at a university (as this study was conducted at two different universities) are bound by ethics rules determined by the university Institutional Research Board (IRB) that protects respondents from abusive or exploitative research practices. Because the IRB at the first university was very nervous about studying sexual minorities in general and defined all nonheterosexuals or people in unconventional relationships as "vulnerable populations," the IRB required me to collect only pseudonyms and did not allow me to keep records of respondents' real names or contact information. While the IRB did this in an effort to protect people's identities, it also made it impossible for me to contact all of the participants in my initial study when I later decided to conduct a longitudinal analysis. The only way I could find previous respondents was to post calls for continued participation on poly Internet sites and via word-of-mouth social networks—both of which would exclude people who no longer interacted with poly communities. The second IRB allowed me to ask for contact information, and I have since been able to track very few people who initially identified as poly for a time and later decided they were no longer polyamorous. Unfortunately, many people who eventually leave a poly lifestyle appear uninterested in spending the time in interviews or possibly fear exposure as a previous polyamorist,[15] and my response rate from former polys is low. This has important implications for my conclusions, as we shall see in part II on families of polyamorists.

Similarly, children are missing from the first two waves of data collection (except for participant observation in which I observed them in community settings but was not allowed to interview them) because I could not attain permission to speak with them. Later, university officials granted me more leeway, and I was finally able to speak to children between five and seventeen years old.[16] Last, the voices of very young children are nearly absent from this book. I did not interview children under five, and interviews with children who were under eight or ten years old tended to be brief and general. Some of them were not aware that they were members of polyamorous families or were unfamiliar with the term *polyamory*, and I did not discuss the term with them unless they brought it up. Most often, I asked general questions about how these young children felt about the adults in their lives and what kinds of things they did, rather than labeling their relationships or introducing terminology.

WHY DO THEY DO POLYAMORY?

Respondents identified six primary reasons for their participation in polyamory, including getting more needs met, more love, sexual variety, family expansion, feeling natural, and rebellion. Most people mentioned multiple reasons why they wanted to have polyamorous relationships.

More Needs Met

By far the most common reason respondents gave for wanting multiple partners was to get more of their needs met in a more humane way. In fact, getting more needs met is such a central trope in polyamorous discussions that we will return to it in chapter 7, "Benefits of Polyamorous Family Life." Polys point out that loading all relational needs on a single relationship is a recipe for disaster. People end up with unmet needs, and others feel pressured to meet partners' needs that they would rather not have to address. For instance, Kevin and Stephanie, a white couple in their mid-thirties, had been married for seven years when Stephanie got sick of what she called Kevin's "constant whining about me depriving him of BDSM (bondage, discipline, sadomasochism). I just wasn't in to it. I had tried it a few times for him but didn't really like it. We went to a club once and it just freaked me out, but he was really excited. We didn't do anything there, but talked a lot about it for months afterwards and ultimately decided that he could go to the club himself and try it out with people who were more in to it." Initially Stephanie was not interested in dating others, and Kevin reported that it took a "frustratingly long time" for him to find dominant female partners (a rarity in high demand in many kinky social settings), so their new resolve was not tested for months. Eventually Kevin was able to "play" (engage in negotiated and sometimes scripted submissive sexual practices such as bondage or impact play, in which the submissive person may be whipped, caned, flogged, or spanked) with dominant women in the scene, though Stephanie viewed Kevin's kinky play as "his other thing, not really sex in a way because he wouldn't have intercourse with them."

Over time, however, as Kevin continued to play with some of the same women in the local kink community and Stephanie reconnected with Joe, an old boyfriend, they became what Stephanie called "real poly or truly poly, instead of poly in the abstract." Stephanie began attending local theater performances regularly with her new beau and realized she was getting needs met that she had not even known she was missing, and Kevin was "thrilled to finally be living out some of my fantasies with women who are enjoying it too." Both found that they were happier with each other as their needs previously unmet were now satiated. Stephanie commented that "I have more appreciation for him [Kevin] now that I am not feeling so much pressure, and I am happier having companionship at the theater, something Kevin always hated but has brought me and Joe back together."

Kevin told me that he and Joe "hang out occasionally and get along fine. We don't have a ton in common, but he seems like a fine guy and the three of us go out for dinner sometimes. I am fine with her seeing him, but would probably not go out of my way to hang out with him otherwise. But he's not problematic or anything, not like I dislike him or anything, we just probably won't end up being best friends because we don't click like that." Similarly, Stephanie did not spend much time with Kevin's "Dommes" (kink community lingo for a dominant woman, used to be called *dominatrix*, but that term has fallen out of favor) because their interactions were in such specialized settings that the women rarely crossed paths with Stephanie.

More Love

Second to getting more of their needs met, poly people mentioned a desire for, and even more importantly a *capacity* for, more love than can be contained in a dyadic (two-person) relationship. For these people, love could come in the form of companionship, attention, conversation, doing special things together, romantic gestures (notes, flowers), sex, shared jokes, and affection. When asked if adding a partner means they love their initial partner less, many polys respond with an analogy that likens gaining a partner to having another child: The arrival of the sibling does not mean that the parents love the first child any less, but that they have a fresh wellspring of love for the new child and continue to love the first child.

Sexual Variety

Not only did people like Stephanie and Kevin end up having different kinds of sex with different kinds of partners, they reported having more sex with different people and taking those experiences back to their primary relationship to invigorate a long-term sexual relationship with new excitement, possibilities, skills, or techniques. While the potential for sexual variety often stands out as the most titillating and important part of polyamory in the general public imagination, it is not often the most compelling reason for people who actually engage in long-term polyamorous relationships. Speaking of his motivations for poly relationships, Zack admitted:

> OK, I guess I am kind of a dirty old man, I like sex a lot. And that was more of a motivating factor at first. But over time it became abundantly clear to me that if I wanted a lot of easy sex poly was not the way to go. Waaaaaaaaay too much talking for that. If I just wanted to get laid by lots of different women all the time then I would have

been a swinger. That's more what that relationship style is for. But poly is so focused on emotions and relationships that sometimes the sex falls by the wayside. But yeah, I like the sex and that is definitely part of it for me. It brings a certain fire to my relationship with Summer when I have been with someone else, and it does the same when she is with someone else too.

Like Zack, Mark reported that he initially focused on sexual variety as a driving force in initiating polyamorous relationships, "but then I grew up a little bit. In fact, over the years, I have grown up a lot and poly has been instrumental in some monumental personal growth for me. The sex is a bonus, but ironically not the main thing for me anymore. If it ever was, really."

Family Expansion

Outside of sexual interactions, many poly folks emphasize the importance of chosen family and multiplication of support. While they often retain contact with their *biolegal* families—or families that are connected through shared parentage and/or marriage—many polyamorists emphasize chosen family as central to their lives. Melody Lupine wanted more children, and her husband, Cristof, was satisfied with the two they already had. Part of the reason Melody was so thrilled when she and Cristof transitioned from a platonic friendship to a romantic polyamorous relationship with their close friend Quentin was that she could have another child, and a "larger family with more love to go around, outside of the framework of one man, one woman." Part II of the book addresses this idea in far greater detail.

It Feels More Natural

For those who experience polyamory as a sexual orientation or innate characteristic, being polyamorous simply feels more natural or comfortable than monogamous relationships. For instance, in response to my query of "Why be poly?" Blake Campo responded: "Because I can not be any other way." He continued:

Whatever it is that's supposed to make people want monogamy, I seem to have been born without it. Even as a kid, it never made

sense to me. On some fundamental level, I have never, ever understood why someone would want monogamy, either personally or for a
partner. The idea of limiting myself to one loving relationship, or
asking a partner to limit herself, just plain doesn't work for me, and it
never has.

Edward Mayfield asserted that polyamory was a

> natural state of being. As far as I'm concerned, everyone is polyamor-
> ous. It's okay, now you start there, you say, okay, what's getting in the
> way? Is jealousy getting in the way? Is your understanding of what
> proper moral behavior, is you know, there are those limitations on
> the behavior, but strictly speaking, everybody wants their needs to be
> met. Everybody, as far as I can tell, is attracted to more than one
> person in their lifetime, and in fact would like to be intimate with
> more than one person in their lifetime, and not just sexually.

People who viewed polyamory as natural often regarded it (and
sometimes bisexuality) as the universal human condition that had been
perverted or tamed by social controls. This rationale served not only to
solidify group cohesion but also to portray those who practiced monogamy as "unnatural" and hence worthy of far greater stigma than the
polyamorists themselves.

Some who saw polyamory as a natural or innate quality were less
sanguine about their involvement. Lucy, a forty-six-year-old white
mother of two, felt some pain in relation to the consequences of her
relationship styles.

> I'm poly because I fall in love with people whether I am in another
> relationship or not, and I can love more than one person at a time
> without (mostly without) feeling jealous or worried. It was painful to
> feel love and passion for people I cared about while I was married,
> and never to be able to do *anything* about it (except cry and write
> poetry) because both I and they were monogamously married. I
> don't want to do that to myself again. If being poly were a
> "choice" . . . I would have dropped it years ago, because of the
> judgment and rejection I have experienced from my family and
> friends. It would not have been worth it.

Others have cultural or social backgrounds that emphasize communality and collective living, and they feel isolated or dislocated when relegated to a dyadic unit cut off or insulated from the larger community or society. Polys in both of these groups report feeling more comfortable in poly relationships than in monogamous relationships, and some emphasize the fact that it is not a choice for them, but they are simply "hardwired this way." Polys who feel most natural in poly relationships are also more likely to see themselves as polyamorous by orientation, something I discuss in greater detail in chapter 1.

Freedom and Rebellion

Other poly people say that polyamory is a choice for them, something they select because it fits with their desire for freedom of self-expression and rebellion against social convention. Shoshanna, a white mother of two in her mid-forties, viewed her engagement in poly relationships as " a way of being I chose . . . I'll admit that my decision to take the choice was a bit political, a bit anti-convention, a bit shit-disturbing." While Shoshanna said she was deeply invested in resisting "the social and gendered constraints of being 'normal' in my relationships," it was not out of mindless revolt, but rather,

> I use the way I live my life as a political tool to some extent, or at least, I want to . . . I resist being ordinary in part, because it traps us and perpetuates inequalities, insecurities and dysfunctions. I like deliberate choice. I like thought-out decisions. That is the real essence of the shit disturbing. I use the term ironically, actually, because I think it's pretty pathetic that taking conscious ownership of what I do and why is often seen as off the grid. I own my relationships, their functioning, my sexuality, its expression and the impact it has on everyone I am in a relationship with, including my kids and parents. I am highly principled, not just rule flaunting.

For polyamorists in this category, following social convention is stifling, and they prefer to customize their relationships to follow their own life course rather than having convention dictate the form of their relationships. They use poly relationships as a statement on social and sexual liberation.

3

POLYAMOROUS COMMUNITIES IN THE UNITED STATES

Polyamorous communities exist online and in person, as well as overlapping with several other communities of nonconformists. Contact among community members is especially important to those who want to form and maintain poly relationships, and those people I spoke with identified the advice and support they received from other community members as crucial to their relational successes. Community contact transmits and reinforces norms and values, provides social support, and supplies a place for polyamorists and their children to "be themselves" without having to constantly explain the presence of multiple partners or parents.

THREE WAVES OF POLYAMORY: A SELECT HISTORY OF NONMONOGAMY IN THE UNITED STATES

Polyamory is a fairly recent addition to a litany of nonmonogamous relationships, some of which have directly influenced the evolution of polyamorous communities. I divide nonmonogamy and polyamory in the United States into three "waves" occurring in the nineteenth, twentieth, and twenty-first centuries.

First Wave: Nineteenth-Century Transcendentalism

There were several groups of people who practiced a multiple-partner relationship style in the United States in the mid to late 1800s, most influenced by the nineteenth-century Transcendental movement. Brook Farm was an "experimental free love community" populated by "Quakers, Shakers, Mormons, and other charismatic leaders who roamed up and down the east coast preaching" a doctrine that "challenged conventional Christian doctrines of sin and human unworthiness."[1]

John Humphrey Noyes founded the Oneida community in 1848. Noyes established a system of "complex marriage" in which "each male was theoretically married to each female, and where each regarded the other as either a brother or a sister."[2] This rejection of monogamous marriage was intended to offer an alternative to "the monogamous relation [which] fostered exclusiveness and selfishness, and worked to counter communism."[3] Children similarly lived together in a communal children's house. Parents were not permitted to show special affection to their own children but were instead mandated to treat all children of the community equally.

Finally, Nashoba was a free-love community established in 1862 by Frances Wright, a wealthy Scottish immigrant. Wright formed a large communal farm, "bringing together both free blacks and whites to work and make love."[4] She opposed the racist trend at the time, and she declared "sexual passion the best source of human happiness."[5]

Second Wave: Twentieth-Century Countercultures

The 1960s and 1970s represented an important period in the evolution of identities that allowed increasing sexual and gender latitude. Feminists included sexual issues such as the repeal of abortion laws and access to safe, legal birth control to their larger agenda of gender equity. Gays and lesbians began to question the hegemony of heterosexuality,[6] and, together with feminists, they exposed gender roles as socially constructed. Transgendered and other transgressive people began to emphasize the performative nature of gender.[7] Bisexuals further destabilized the blend of gender and sexuality by minimizing the importance of their romantic partners' genders.[8] Finally, social and economic conditions contributed to an increase in autonomy for women and sexual minorities, especially gays and lesbians. Industrialization, shrinking families, and the separation of sexuality from procreation enabled women to bear fewer children and gays and lesbians to develop urban enclaves.[9] Polyamory evolved as a direct result of the sexual revolution and intertwined with the alternative sexual forms previously discussed, especially the bisexual and free love movements. Like other aspects of the polyamorous community, the history of the movement has some points of contention.

Communes

One form of countercultural group was the commune. The community movement, which had declined in the United States during the late nineteenth century, reemerged in the form of communes in 1960s and 1970s. This second iteration maintained a focus on creating a chosen family for people who were "establishment dropouts, disillusioned with the dominant lifestyles in America; they are people who believe they can find a better way of life in a group living experience with like-minded persons."[10] Communes often emphasized the value of intimate relationships, personal growth, spiritual rebirth, and cooperation over competition, return to nature, and rebellion against the establishment. Many communities included some form of atypical sexuality, from celibacy to free love,[11] though only a minority of contemporary communes endorsed sexually nonexclusive relationships.[12]

Specifically polyamorous communes evolved in the late 1960s and early 1970s. John and Barbara Williamson established the Sandstone community in Los Angeles after the Kirkridge Sexuality Conferences that "served to network polyamorous clergy, researchers, writers, and artists on the East coast."[13] Sandstone was "the encounter-group oriented love community in Topanga Canyon," California, and it included such eminent counterculturalists as Betty Dodson and Sally Binford.[14]

Kerista, possibly the most influential nonmonogamous, protopolyamorous intentional community, was based in the San Francisco Bay Area between 1971 and 1991. Strassberg noted:

> During the twenty-year existence of the community, the approximately twenty-five adult members lived either in separate group marriages or in a single group marriage . . . [Kerista] was based on an

experimental lifestyle that included group marriage, shared parenting, total economic sharing, a group growth process, and a utopian plan for improving life around the world by replicating their model of community living.[15]

Members owned and operated a computer sales business. During her tenure there, Ryam Nearing reported living in a community that attempted to provide emotional support for everyone. Nearing participated in seeking a Keristan vision which "started with twelve but later amped it up to twenty-four adults per family in their ideal—the goal they wanted to aim for."[16]

"Multilateral" Marriage and Swinging

Two more countercultural groups involved "multilateral" or group marriage and swinging. Research into these nonmonogamous relationships peaked in the early 1970s. By that time, the sexual revolution had popularized sexual experimentation, and the concepts of open and group marriages had gained notoriety. American culture was more sexually permissive than ever before, and the specter of AIDS had not yet destroyed the playful sense of sexual experimentation. Researchers such as Constantine and Constantine[17] studied those involved in "multilateral marriages," which they defined as "three or more partners, each of whom considers him/herself to be married (or committed in a functionally analogous way) to more than one of the other partners." Smith and Smith[18] compiled studies of "sexual alternatives in marriage" in an edited collection that examined such diverse topics as comarital sex (the open incorporation of extramarital sex into marital unions),[19] group sex,[20] infidelity,[21] and group marriage.[22]

Research on swinging similarly flourished in the sexually adventurous 1960s and 1970s, documenting new trends in extramarital or comarital sexual involvement.[23] Studies examined swingers' race and ethnicity,[24] social class,[25] education,[26] and political perspectives.[27] This research created a profile of a swinger as a "white, middle to upper middle class person in his or her late thirties who is fairly conventional in all ways except for her or his lack of religious participation/identification and participates in swinging."[28] Once the sexual revolution collided with the spread of AIDS and other sexually transmitted infections in the 1980s, research on sexually nonexclusive relationships dwindled. Although very few such studies were published during the 1980s and 1990s, the practice of nonmonogamous relationships endured.

Support Groups

Informal and organized prototypical polyamorous support groups began to spread in the 1970s, the best known of which were Family Synergy in Los Angeles and Family Tree in Boston. Inspired by Robert Heinlein's *Stranger in a Strange Land*,[29] Oberon Zell-Ravenheart founded the Church of All Worlds and its related Ravenheart clan, still influential in the polyamorous movement today. Individuals started organizations focused on polyamory or polyfidelity, such as Ryam Nearing's Polyfidelitous Educational Productions (PEP), a group in Denver called Beyond Monogamy that met regularly and published an edited volume, and Deborah Anapol's IntiNet. Nearing and Anapol later teamed up to create *Loving More* magazine (which subsequently became Nearing's solo project and has since then transitioned through several editors) that published articles, poetry, and personal advertisements for, by, and about polyamorous people.

Third Wave: Impact of the Internet

Contemporary research indicates that alternative sexual styles such as polyamory have increased with the advent of Internet technology, which facilitates communication between geographically disparate people seeking support for alternative relationships.[30] In recent years, the Internet has proved an especially important site for community building among marginalized populations. Sexual nonconformists have populated the Internet in droves, forming personal and sexual connections online.[31] The impact of the worldwide web on polyamorous (and other sexual minority) communities would be difficult to overstate. From dating or discussing jealousy to asking for advice, much polyamorous relating occurs "online." The extensive network of Internet communication has spawned an impressive number of polyamorous websites.

While polyamorous websites are too numerous to adequately list here, I have included some of the more important ones as examples of online community. Lovemore.com is *Loving More* magazine's website. It includes not only a bulletin board but also a chat room, frequently asked questions (FAQ), stories, advice, events, "the love list" (a summary of conversations that transpired on the electronic discussion board that was emailed to list subscribers), and personal ads for those seeking others to engage in polyamorous relationships. Yahoo lists over one hundred polyamorous groups by region and interest, accessible through their "romance and relationships" section or simply by entering the key search word *polyamory*.

Alt.polyamory contains an extensive list of polyamorous information, including six different FAQ pages, a glossary of acronyms, abbreviations, and new words found on polyamorous sites, a list of polyamorous resources including fiction, nonfiction, music, movies, "poly-friendly" professionals such as mental health counselors and ministers willing to perform group marriages, art, and paraphernalia such as T-shirts and mugs. Alt.polyamory also hosts numerous topical email lists for specific subgroups including activists, parents, triads, and those seeking intentional community. Those who wish to post or read personal ads are directed to alt.personals, soc.personals, or alt.personals.poly. The "poly ring" is for members only, and it links diverse polyamorous sites across the web. PolyMatchMaker.com lists personal ads for those seeking polyamorous relationships. It, too, is open to members only, though memberships are free. Finally, numerous polyamorists' personal websites include stories of their polyamorous lifestyles, links to other pages, pictures, poetry, journal entries, artwork, information about upcoming events, and calls to activism.

Polyamorists also link to other related, but not explicitly polyamorous, websites. Janesguide.com, a guide to alternative-sex-oriented sites on the web, is a favorite among web-savvy polyamorists, as is LiveJournal.com—a free site that allows writers to create journals online and choose to make their writing available to select others or to anyone visiting the site. LiveJournal lists over one hundred relevant "community" matches and over 1,300 users interested in polyamory. Sites that contain information about swinging may overlap with polyamorous sites, and the communities share personal ads at www.altdot.com. The polyamorous presence on the web is diverse and serves as a vital component of community formation and participation.

CHARACTERISTICS OF POLYAMOROUS COMMUNITIES

Polyamorous communities exist in both a geographic sense and online. Local or geographic communities vary tremendously in their level of organization and political involvement. Smaller communities tend to have very little organization and are virtually nonexistent as political entities. Larger communities seem far better organized, and members are often involved in the politics of polyamory. Community politics happen among activists and longer-term polyamorists who have known each other for many years and for whom polyamory is a central component of their identities. These longer-term polyamorists are the same people who have evolved into community leaders: some are leaders of their local groups and others leaders of the loosely defined national movement. Leaders often live in established centers of polyamorous activity, and new centers grow up around leaders who relocate to new areas. Some who used to be leaders and grew tired of the media attention and community activism have withdrawn from leadership positions.

Geographic Distribution of Polyamory

Polyamory flourishes primarily in urban population centers. The California Bay Area is home to numerous interlocking groups and several nationally recognized leaders. Several more leaders live in Southern California, with its less organized and more cellular polyamorous communities. Boston, New York, Seattle, and Washington, D.C., are also centers for polyamorous activity.

The Hawaiian Islands, another nexus of polyamorous life, each host their own individual polyamorous communities that vary by size and degree of public acknowledgment. Jane and Sam consider themselves (and were considered so by some) national leaders, as well as leaders of a Hawaiian Island polyamorous community. They characterize their local polyamorous community as the following:

> Most of the poly folks around here are hidden. They don't identify themselves as poly, just live life with multiple relationships. The missionaries have done a good job [preaching monogamy]. Oahu is a different scene. There's a much larger population of polys there.

Both the West and East coasts of the United States emphasize polyamory and sex positivity,[32] while the Midwest hosts a more conservative
community focused primarily on polyfidelity.

Urban and Rural Distribution of Polyamory

Typical of sexual minorities in general, polyamorists who lived near
large population centers seemed more successful at finding acceptance
and others with whom to practice polyamory. Those in rural settings
were isolated[33] and often traveled to nearby urban areas or sought
support, advice, and long-distance relationships online in polyamorous
cybercommunities.

Bethany and Chad, a white, polyamorous married couple in their
mid-thirties and late fifties, respectively, lived in a small agricultural
town in the Midwest, roughly a seven-hour drive from a large population center. They tended hogs for a large agribusiness, working long
hours to support their five children (two of whom were Chad's from a
previous marriage). Even so, they barely had enough money to pay the
rent every month, and their second car was repossessed when they
could not make the payments, leaving them with a pickup truck as the
sole form of transportation for the family of seven. They could not
afford Internet access to make contact with online polyamorous communities, and they subsequently suffered intense feelings of isolation,
distress, and loneliness.

Internet access was financially out of reach for Bethany and Chad, so
their primary contact with the polyamorous community was during an
annual polyamorous campout several hundred miles from their home.
Bethany confided to me that she felt "at home" during the gatherings in
a way she usually did not experience in other parts of her life. "I feel
like I can be myself here, not like at home. I cry all the way to [a distant
town on their way home] every time we leave one of these things."
While Bethany and Chad sought polyamorous community as a way to
feel "at home," they were distinct from the majority of community
members in many ways. Not only did they live in a rural area but also
their agricultural occupations paid little, distinguishing them from the
majority of other polyamorists, who were middle and upper-middle
class and tended to be able to afford to socialize online frequently.

Online Communities

While online communities provide education for members of the public, their primary function is to allow polyamorists (and other sexual minorities) to mingle in cybercommunities. Previously isolated people find others on the web, and community becomes redefined as an affective, information-based link, free of geographical boundaries. Virtual communities offer a substitute for live social gatherings as well as a way for those separated geographically to establish a cohesive community identity. Online mingling occurs in a number of forums: bulletin boards, chat rooms, email lists, and personal websites, with a variety of information including frequently asked question pages (FAQs), journal entries, photographs, or directions to homes for polyamorous gatherings.

The social structure of online polyamorous communities contains a variety of types of members and appeared to be similar to other online communities.[34] People are occasionally harsh to one another, but more often they offer support, advice, and solace. For those willing to engage in long-distance relationships, online communities offer a much larger pool of potential dating partners. People interacting with each other on poly websites expect each other to have a certain degree of web savvy—most web users have pseudonyms and often control access to particularly identifying information. Web communities are often cohesive enough to establish a collective sense of identity and thus can mutually agree to ostracize someone who violates community norms, effectively policing their own boundaries.

FUNCTIONS OF POLYAMOROUS COMMUNITIES

Poly people often emphasized the vital importance of community to the health of their relationships and individual happiness. To that end, polyamorous peoples' associations fulfilled a number of functions of polyamory. Bringing people together entailed introducing them to the local or cyber community where they would find a selection of dating partners.

Bringing People Together

Community is especially important for bringing together polys and other sexual minorities who are marginalized from society because they provide role models, a pool of potential partners, and assistance in a world where nonconformists are often targets of stigma and disdain. Community membership offers many benefits, and one of the most important is the ability to conceive of an alternative identity in which the unusual characteristic is acceptable and the support to take on that identity and maintain it. Polyamorous people routinely seek to join or create communities with like-minded others.

Some people search out or stumble upon a polyamorous subculture (usually online, but occasionally in person), and others are recruited by lovers or potential lovers hoping to involve them in poly relationships. Many people discover the idea of multiple relationships through science fiction,[35] and some establish multiple-partner relationships first and come to identify as polyamorous when they later discover the term.

Learning the Term *Polyamory*

For some polyamorists, introduction to the term *polyamory* was a monumental occurrence. People who were previously isolated in their desire to experience multiple partnerships talked about feeling as if a new world had opened to them when they found out about the term. For these folks, a relationship style that was previously inconceivable suddenly became plausible when they heard the term and discovered the associated community and identity. This mirrors Weinberg's[36] findings that, for some people, the "discovery of the category [bisexual] in fact existed was a turning point" in how they came to think of themselves as bisexual.

Sybil, a white woman in her late thirties, described her feelings when she first learned the term *polyamory* from someone who had listed it in her Yahoo! profile.

> I wrote to her and asked what the heck is that? She wrote back and explained it and I was like *oh my god*! You mean you can really *do* that? There are other people who feel this way! I didn't know people actually did that—*oh my god*! I walked around for the rest of the day

just amazed, like holy shit! I didn't know anyone else who was poly yet then, but just knowing it existed made me feel so free.

Sybil explained that she had always desired relationships with multiple partners but had never done so openly because she did not think it possible within the constraints of monogamous society. She had been in few truly monogamous relationships, and most of them had ended when she was caught cheating.

Finding the term *polyamory* was not as earth shattering for other people who were already familiar with the concept of nonmonogamy. Joya explained that "I started out feeling like I had options and I don't know where those, that came from. Perhaps being an avid sci fi reader as a young person, where people were saying your relationships did not necessarily have to look one way."

Others were already conducting polyamorous relationships when they became aware of the term. Edward Mayfield reported finding himself involved in a polyamorous relationship, and then realizing there was not only a term but also a community of people who lived their lives this way and talked to each other about it.

> We [he and his wife, Monique] met this other couple. I was infatuated by the woman, and Monique seemed to like the guy just fine and, you know, I'm scratching my head a little bit. What's happening here? And we discuss this and we actually went into a relationship. It seemed right . . . and we ended up spending a lot of time with them eventually because of some external stuff and eventually moved in with them for a time and actually stayed and found a place with them and actually moved to [another state] with them. I don't think we were calling it anything in particular but we got involved. It just seemed the right thing to do at the time.

The Mayfields had no plan, no label for their alternative relationship form. They simply realized they were in love and it "seemed the right thing to do."

Others became aware of the concept of polyamory through their social networks. Morgan Majek had heard about polyamory through a Pagan group with whom she worshipped regularly. She had not considered herself polyamorous until

I met a man named Derek. He started coming to the meetings, and I just clicked instantly and was physically attracted and mentally attracted. He's Pagan and we were able to just talk very easily and communicate very easily. And we started hanging out with each other as friends and then we started falling in love and it just happened over about five or six months. And then we discussed it, Derek and I, because our feelings were getting really, really strong and we discussed trying to begin a relationship because he had heard of polyamory and been to the [Internet] sites and read about it. And so we decided we were gonna tell our spouses.

Morgan's initial dim awareness of polyamory suddenly became much more important once she found herself simultaneously in love with Derek and her husband, Carl. Finding a poly community with a specific word helped not only to label and solidify polyamory as a personal identity but also it became something Morgan and Edward could do or be—a poly person with an identity based on the mutual relationship style of community members.[37]

Selection of Dating Partners

Polyamorous communities not only provide their members a group of like-minded people from whom to seek potential partners but also have useful information about those people as well. Much like gays, lesbians, and other sexual minorities,[38] polyamorists often encounter difficulty finding other polys, or monogamists willing to explore polyamory. Polyamorous communities offer members access to one another: potential partners that they can depend on to be (in varying degrees) familiar with community norms and values and open to the possibility of multiple-partner relationships.

Polyamorists often found their partners' romantic relationships with nonpolyamorous people problematic, because the nonpolyamorists' ignorance of community norms often negatively impacted the primary polyamorous relationship. These relationships were laden with all of the problems associated with newbie relationships, as well as the additional challenge of incorporating ostensibly monogamous partners. Sometimes a monogamist and a polyamorist could have a clash of the paradigms, with each attempting to get the other to convert. Other people found the lack of common norms problematic. Louise Amore discussed her qualms regarding Max's (her husband at the time) relationship with Elana:

> It was difficult for a lot of reasons. One of which was that I didn't know her. She was married and cheating on her husband, and that just didn't, she just didn't understand how important, she wasn't willing to talk to me. Whereas people who are polyamorous understand the need to talk to each other. . . . If I don't know who he's involved with it's very hard for me, because I don't trust them. . . . Max very much fell in love with this woman and it was, and because she was, I don't like her. She thinks that cheating is a game and she plays with people's lives, and it surprised me that Max would want to get involved with someone like that. . . . I didn't expect her to know our rules or to even respect them because she doesn't respect the rules of her own marriage. How's she gonna respect mine?

Not only were polyamorous community members socialized into shared norms and values such as honesty and communication, they also tended to be more of a "known quantity" as well.

Once polyamorists entered a community and were "road tested" by a number of relationships, other community members gained information about them that allowed more informed decisions regarding the possibility of dating those people. Marilyn, a white woman in her early thirties attending a bisexual coffeehouse gathering in the Bay Area, discussed what she called "partnersharing," the practice of "checking out" partners of friends. "If I see someone who has had a lot of drama in successive relationships then it gives me a red flag, not like I judge them, but it is something to look out for." She gained this valuable information through her interactions with overlapping bisexual and polyamorous communities in the Bay Area.

Assistance

Polyamorous communities not only helped poly people find each other but they also created a community forum where people could help each other. The quality of social interaction in close-knit poly communities struck me as quite similar to people who share the same church—they may not see each other every day but interact frequently enough that they know that if something happens there is a group of people ready to help them and who they would help in turn. Because most poly people either don't practice any religion or practice an uncommon form of religion (Paganism, Buddhism, and Unitarian Universalism are the most popular), poly communities can provide them with a level of group cohesion and mutual aid that they would otherwise find hard to come by without membership in a close-knit synagogue, church, or temple.

Financial Assistance

Polyamorists give each other financial assistance in times of need, especially if it is a need created as a result of a polyamorous relationship. Their local poly community rallied around a couple in the San Francisco Bay Area when they were fired from a local church and lost their employee housing because their polyamorous relationships became public knowledge. Personally and financially devastated, the unemployed couple sent a message to their local polyamorous email list pleading, "We need help, please!" A list member found them free housing (temporarily) in exchange for painting the apartment. Although being outed as polyamorous cost them their jobs and home, their involvement with the local polyamorous community provided them with assistance to ease the effects of discrimination.

Poly people routinely helped each other. Melody Lupine rented a large house that became a center for people seeking connections with the local polyamorous community:

> Many people have come to live with me and they don't have much money to begin with and with the move and a big expense like that, I won't charge them the first month's rent when they're staying with me, but they know once they get back on their feet, they pay me back. So, and I've helped out. Cristof's (one of her husbands) helped me out and I've helped him out, vice versa. There's an ebb and flow with it . . . so it's taught me a lot about how to do that being in a polyamorous community.

Melody connected her generosity directly with her experiences of reciprocity within her local poly community. Things did not always work out well for Melody, however. At least once, people who were living with her moved out in the middle of the night without paying her the rent they owed. They were new to polyamory and had not yet been socialized into the community norms of generosity and honesty. The majority of the polys I met appeared more than willing to offer emotional support, and maybe even financial assistance as well depending on the circumstances.

The national polyamorous community rallied around April Divilbliss when she faced losing custody of her child because she was in a poly relationship.[39] Divilbliss lived for a time in a triadic relationship with two men, neither of whom was the father of her child. When the child's paternal grandmother discovered this, she sought legal custody of her grandchild. Divilbliss moved out of her triadic household and lived alone with her child, but the action satisfied neither her ex mother-in-law nor the courts. She reached out to polyamorous communities[40] who fueled her custody battle with financial and emotional support, but she eventually lost custody of her child.[41] The national polyamorous community collectively viewed Divilbliss's loss as a defeat any nonmonogamous family might have to endure.[42]

Emotional Assistance

Even more important than financial assistance, polyamorous community members provided each other emotional assistance in the form of empathy, advice, and a new frame of reference to normalize their lifestyle. Penny and Marcus, both white peace activists in their late forties, were married for twenty-three years. They were very close with Nick and Leah—another white peace activist couple in their late forties— and for fifteen years they helped to raise Nick and Leah's son, Connor. After years of spending three to five days a week together for family activities and socializing, Penny and Nick fell in love. They approached their respective spouses to discuss their feelings. Nick had erroneously anticipated that Leah would welcome Penny as his future lover, because he and Leah had been in a quad years before meeting Penny and Marcus. Instead, Penny said that "Leah freaked out. It was a huge trainwreck; we still have not recovered."

Penny explained that the peace community rallied around Leah, telling her, "Of course this level of distress is appropriate and how kind and understanding she is to put up with our [Penny and Nick's] terrible philandering." Penny complained that no one in the peace community was telling Leah, "You know, this level of jealousy is really problematic, maybe you should seek some help in dealing with this out-of-control insecurity." Feeling ostracized, Penny grieved the absence of support from her usual sources in the peace community whom she had known and socialized with for many years. She attributed this to being viewed as "The baaaaad girl!" Penny expressed her gratitude to polyamorous community members who offered their support during this difficult period. "I am so glad to find you people. I feel like less of a freak now that I know there are actually people who *do* this. You guys are from the home planet!" Penny's portrayal of other polyamorists as "from the home planet" underlined how thoroughly estranged she felt from her customary social surroundings and how comforted she felt with like-minded people.

Support group meetings offered a forum for polys to discussed their complex relationships in a safe environment where they could expect understanding rather than condemnation. Carlie, a thirty-five-year-old white educator and mother of two, came to a support meeting and tearfully related "the disaster my life has become" since the relationship between the two men she loved degenerated into bitterness and jealousy. She responded to the sympathy and advice offered by the group, "Thanks guys! I needed to hear something else from people besides, 'well, what did you expect to happen, you little slut?'" Members of this support group, like others in polyamorous communities, offered not only advice and support but also a way to normalize the difficult life events in poly life as unpleasant but average family difficulties.

THE (MOSTLY UNWRITTEN) SOCIAL RULES IN POLY COMMUNITIES

In sociology we frequently talk about *norms*, or the unwritten social rules specific to a society or social group that guide and limit behaviors. When someone breaks the norms and does something unusual, they are being *deviant*. The two concepts are intertwined—norms define deviance as out of bounds, and deviance contrasts with normative behavior to highlight the differences between the two. In other words, we know what is socially correct precisely because we know what is socially incorrect.[43] When people break social rules for behavior they are subject to *stigma*, or the negative social judgment that comes with having a difference that is "discrediting" and "spoils" the person's reputation.[44]

Poly communities have their own norms that establish guidelines for behaviors and interactions among poly folks, and newbies (people new to polyamory) learn the norms from role models who demonstrate and explain community social conventions. As is true of most groups, poly community norms are founded on idealized visions of polyamory, and some people are not always able to live up to the high standards of the ideal.

Morning Glory Zell-Ravenheart's foundational "A Bouquet of Lovers" (or "Rules of the Road")[45] provides guidelines to structure polyamorous relationships. While not formally enforced, many second-wave polyamorists read and discussed the rules of the road at support groups or social gatherings, and over time they have permeated the community so that they have become collective sensibilities.

Poly communities generally value honesty above anything else, and it is the single most important norm that underlies the others.[46] Long-term polys expect each other to be honest, and they explain the importance of the norm by linking honesty to trust, without which poly relationships do not work. Lying leads to distrust, which undermines the emotional safety that is only possible when people trust each other. Online and in support groups, polys regularly discuss ways to effectively and humanely maintain honest relationships. While those who fail to follow strict codes of honesty are stigmatized, they are not dealt with very harshly because nearly everyone has lied to someone at least once. If the liar later tells the truth and makes amends, polys will generally be understanding of the lapse, though repeat offenders are stigmatized more severely than first timers.

Another key poly community norm requires that everyone in a given relationship be bound by the same rules, regardless of gender: men and women have equal access to outside lovers within the same negotiated agreement. Generally, community members frown on relationships that allow one member access to outside lovers but deny another the same liberty.[47] A related norm involves the idea of equal power between and among relationship partners. Community rhetoric supports equality and casts power sharing as its central component. Some polyamorists successfully attain this idealized norm, and others struggle to achieve it or simply have an inequitable balance of power.

Role Models

Consensual nonmonogamy is so uncommon in the United States that most people in poly relationships do not have easy access to relationship role models in their own families of origin or even popular media. Polyamorous communities provide that role modeling and demonstrate patterns that other families can mimic if they prove useful. Spending time with seasoned polyamorists helps newbies find the role models so essential in this potentially complex and fluid relationship style. These role models give newbies an alternative reference group,[48] teaching new relationship skills and providing a different frame of reference from conventional monogamous society.

Role models also transmitted information and relationship skills, and discovery of a polyamorous subculture improved some people's relationship skills and offered a fresh perspective on their past and current relationships. Louise Amore, a thirty-seven-year-old photographer and mother of three, said she learned new relationship tools through contact with local and online polyamorous communities. These tools helped to improve her relationship with her husband, Max, a forty-one-year-old father of three and computer programmer. Louise and Max had originally agreed to an open marriage, but "we didn't really know what we were doing." They initially attempted a "don't ask, don't tell" approach in which they could establish outside relationships as long as the other remained unaware. Louise explained that she was uncomfortable with the arrangement:

> During that time I was the only one who did see someone and I didn't like lying. Again, it just didn't seem much different than being monogamous and lying and cheating, because I still wasn't being honest about what I was doing. And so that lasted just a few weeks and I said I can't do this, and so for eight years we were monogamous. And it opened up after we found the Internet and when we found there were other people out there, we weren't the only weirdoes. And from there it progressed into—we finally, about two years ago found the polyamory groups and there was actually a word for who we were and the way we related to people.

Louise's discovery of an online polyamorous community offered her an alternative way to think about her relationship with Max, and relating with other polyamorists gave both Louise and Max the skills to support their new relationship style.

People who had established multiple-partner relationships in isolation from other nonmonogamists would sometimes rewrite their social histories once they started socializing with poly communities. Bruce, a man in his mid-forties, expressed his glee that

> I ain't no cheating, low-life horn dog no more! [laughing] I was poly the whole time. I had no idea how to ask for my needs with other partners to be met, so I did it behind their backs. Now I am honest about it and it's much better.

Discovery of the polyamorous community assisted Bruce in rehabilitating himself from "low-life horn dog" to a *poly* person with an identity based in an ethical community. Redemption of the past[49] allowed Bruce and others like him to recast past mistakes, and also provided a welcome rationale for polyamorous activities that conflicted with the social mandates of a culture that celebrates monogamy. Poly socializing provided not only role models but also an alternative moral and emotional framework in which to understand their own actions as beneficial to themselves, their partners, and their relationships as well.

Polys who did not have access to role models often said they felt adrift, alone, and confused. Steve, a white man in his mid-forties, who had practiced polyamory intermittently since his late teens (though he did not call it polyamory until he heard the word in his early forties), recounted his teenage involvement with a group of friends engaged in what he retrospectively called "the poly experiment." Steve was the de facto leader of the group, though he said:

> I wasn't mature enough to handle that level of complexity in my first attempt at poly. There were no adult role models for us to follow; we were trying to create this thing by reading *The Harrad Experiment*.[50] A few people got majorly burned. We were in so far over our heads; we had no idea what we were doing.

Lack of community and attendant role models contributed to the failure of that particular "experiment." Steve, however, did not abandon his multiple-relational practices, and instead he refined it, partially through contact with the polyamorous community.

"Hubs" as Role Models

Hubs—compact geographic centers of polyamorous activity—emerged in poly communities, frequently forming around an extended family, or a couple with many lovers, with the resources to gather community and host events. When Jana Founder's moresome melded with Melody Lupine's triad, they created a combined family of eight adults and four children. Six of the adults resided within a five-block radius, and the other two visited periodically. The combined physical space, increased number of family members, and numerous ancillary lovers and friends created a hub for local community social events and support groups. The magnetic pull of the hub drew other people who were considering or practicing polyamory, who then remained in the area in part because of the quality of community available. This created a self-perpetuating cycle in which the presence of an organized community attracted others seeking polyamorous fellowship, strengthening the existing local community.

Within fifteen miles of the Founder/Lupine hub, Louise Amore created an additional social hub when she opened her home to polyamorous gatherings and organized polyamorous outings such as camping trips. Similar hubs formed in the California Bay Area around Evelyn and Mark Coach, the Wyss family, and the Ravenheart clan composed of long-term national community leaders and their many ancillary lovers.

Hub members tended to emphasize polyamory as a core aspect of their personal identities. Polyamory was a central identity characteristic to members of the Founder/Lupine hub, and similar community leaders. These leaders published books and magazines on polyamory, conducted radio and television interviews, organized conferences, managed email lists and websites, and acted as a clearing house of information for members of the general public seeking assistance or information surrounding polyamorous issues. The sheer amount of time they spent discussing and writing about polyamory made it a key component of their lives. Add to that the time they spent practicing polyamory, holding house meetings, and discussing feelings with lovers, and there was little time left for other things. The centrality of polyamory to people's identities tended to wane with members' increased social distance from the center of the hub.

When a hub family broke up it usually had a considerable impact on surrounding community members. Losing the social territory previously defined as polyamorous meant fewer places to gather, less emotional and financial support, and lower chances of meeting potential partners. Role models and friends became more difficult to find and existing relationships more difficult to maintain. People questioned the longevity of their own relationships when a hub family, which had served as a key role model for the local community, broke up. The ancillary lovers of the hub sometimes drifted away, and others considered becoming monogamous.

Stigma Against Monogamists

Ironically, focusing on honesty and self-knowledge as key to poly identity allows polys to reverse the stigma onto monogamous people the polys see as narrow-minded or stuck, as Jeffrey, a white male in his mid-forties, put it:

> Not all people in monogamous relationships, I'm sure some are good, but in some of them people are cowering or cheating because they don't have the balls it takes to be honest about it. I know, I used to be one of them, and then I grew up (laughing). It's kinda true though, that being poly made me "put on my big boy pants" as my wife loves to say.

Jeffrey shared the common poly community view of subtly (and sometimes not so subtly) portraying monogamous people as small and grasping, too weak to face the self-awareness boot camp that poly family life can be. Poly people, in this sentiment, are more evolved, stronger, and self-realized than mere monogamists.

Polyamorous Deviance

In the discipline of sociology, the term *deviance* means simply being outside of the norm. Theoretically, the sociological term does not have the negative connotations it carries in conventional society, although some scholars doubt that "kinder and gentler" view of deviance.[51] While polyamorists live by a wider range of norms than that found in traditional monogamous society, sometimes they break even their own unique social rules. A number of offenses qualify as deviant among poly community members, and polys usually deal with them through gossip and subtle social pressure. Such deviance rarely erupts into open social conflict.

Cheating

Dating married people without the monogamous spouse's knowledge is generally severely stigmatized among poly folks, and frequently it results in social censure and a damaged reputation. Any form of deceit is largely frowned upon, as it violates the fundamental community ideals of communication and honesty. Even so, some polyamorists lie to each other with surprising regularity, and dishonesty is a constant topic of discussion in support groups and online forums. Possibly the most stigmatized forms of deception involves failure to disclose STIs or breaking safer-sex agreements. Community members often went to great lengths to educate themselves regarding STIs, and they painstakingly negotiated safer-sex agreements to protect themselves from exposure and to prevent transmission to others. Breaches in safer-sex agreements are considered especially problematic because they can pose serious risks to fluid-bonded partners.

Ironically, people in polyfidelitous relationships sometimes cheat on their spice by having sexual relationships outside of the approved group. There are a number of reasons people cheat within polyamorous relationships. A desire for drama, the adrenaline rush that accompanies the spy games of a clandestine relationship, the potential to gain power over another partner by keeping secrets, or even to avoid the inevitable complexities of their partners knowing of one another can all be motivations to cheat, for polys and infidelitous serial monogamists. The Sommers polyfidelitous quad was composed of Frank and Georgia Some and Linda and Marlin Mers, two previously monogamously married white couples who had merged to form a larger family unit, and they eventually broke up over Marlin's infidelity with a former girlfriend. The "other woman" did not wish to join the quad, claiming that she was monogamous and unable (or unwilling, depending on whose opinion you followed) to be in a polyfidelitous relationship. Linda, whom Marlin had legally married years before joining the quad, wondered aloud in a support group meeting how this woman, who was having a relationship with a "very married man," could still call herself monogamous.

The Sommers quad eventually dissolved, ostensibly because of the infidelity, though members mentioned other contributing problems. Marlin was mildly stigmatized by the polyamorous community at large and was especially harshly stigmatized by Linda, who gossiped in person and ranted online about his many alleged personal and sexual inadequacies. Even with Linda's hurt and anger, Marlin still attended polyamorous functions with Georgia and appeared to retain a fairly positive standing in the community. Some people found Linda's tirades over the top and stigmatized her for being too harsh, either by gossiping to each other about Linda or responding to her online diatribes. Other former quad members also remained involved in the community and tried to avoid each other with varying degrees of success. Among poly community members, the main method of punishing people who misbehaved was gossip, and offenders were rarely ostracized.

Joya Starr told me about a time she experienced polyamorous cheating:

> I felt exploited by being open to my partners being in other relationships but that not being reciprocated. Like they were uncomfortable with my relationships or say that they wanted to be in a trio but they continuously became involved with people who were monogamous and wanted to undermine my relationship with my partner. And that's been—more jealousy has come up around that than anything else ever for me. And I find it particularly annoying when polyamory is out as a possibility, on the table, part of how we relate to each other, but they really prefer to cheat. They want to have their relationship but not wanting to reciprocate that relationship for me so they hide that they're involved with somebody else as if I'm stupid. . . . You've got this poly surface, but with that energy of cheating inside of it. And I found out that some people just love that and it's not poly. They love that cheating stuff. . . . I think it was that balance of power where that was part of the turn-on was the hiding part.

Joya, like many community members, felt that lying and cheating in a polyamorous relationship was "not poly," although it was common enough to indicate that it is a poly practice, even if it is not poly philosophy.

Double Standard

Another way in which polys would break the unwritten community rules is when one person wants free access to multiple lovers themselves but finds it difficult to "allow" their partner(s) to have additional lovers as well. When the double standard is overt, people come right out and say, "I don't want you seeing anyone else, but I want to be able to see these other people." At other times it is more subtle, with one of the partners saying, "I am fine with you having other lovers," and then vetoing every candidate for one reason or another, in effect depriving their partner of other lovers while pretending otherwise. This double standard goes against the community philosophy that recommends the same rules for everyone and is wary of relationships that give one partner more latitude than another. People with a double standard were stigmatized, and such relationships often self-destructed. The double standard was not gender specific, and both men and women occasionally wished to restrain a partner from seeing others while enjoying multiple partners themselves. Melody Lupine detailed a relationship she had had with a man in which his girlfriend had a double standard regarding sexual involvement with others:

> She broke up with him and then called him and wanted him back. He had gotten into another relationship and that became real insecure for her and she didn't like it. It brought up a lot of her issues, and all of a sudden he started looking better and fears of hers came up. But what had happened, there's a double standard with her now. It's okay for her to be polyamorous, but she doesn't like that he is, and doesn't like that he's in a relationship with me.

Community members often stigmatized people who held on to the double standard; not only did it violate cherished community norms of equality and ethical treatment but also such noxious jealousy kept the person with the double standard from participating in the highly esteemed community ideal of compersion. Double-standard relationships should not be confused with poly-mono relationships, in which both partners have explicit permission to engage in outside relationships but only one of them feels the desire to do so.

THE IMPORTANCE OF COMMUNICATION

Communication and honesty are such important aspects of polyamorous life that it is difficult to overemphasize them. Together, they are the most popular coping mechanisms that assist polyamorists in dealing with the potential difficulties in their complex relationship style. Polyamorists routinely face the possibility of jealousy, hurt feelings, and miscommunication among many partners. While monogomists experience these same difficulties in their own relationships, the increased number of people in polyamorous relationships multiplies the opportunities for miscommunication significantly. Polys developed a number of techniques to deal with these potential pitfalls. One such mechanism was *radical honesty*, a practice of being completely honest in all situations, even when it was not "nice" or convenient.[52] Many long-term polys practiced and even sought training in Nonviolent Communication (NVC)[53] techniques, such as listening compassionately to the other person while they are speaking instead of preparing mental notes for a rebuttal, subverting the desire to argue by calmly repeating what the other person said back to them to make sure everyone shares the same understanding, and speaking in "*I* statements."

Poly community members also value persistence and the ability to tolerate conflict, in large part because the humane practice of those traits contributes to effective communication. Morgan Majek commented, "I'm willing to work through things, so I'll just talk things to death and work through 'em." Morgan felt her relationship with her husband, Carl, had improved since they became polyamorous, primarily because

> It really opened up communication between us. Because we've been together for nine years and that was my biggest complaint about him was you don't talk to me . . . And it really opened up communication between us. So it created pain, but it really just helped us to learn how to be completely honest and communicate. And so it benefited us.

Discussing painful feelings such as jealousy or insecurity can take tremendous fortitude, and establishing schedules that allow many lovers time with one another required adept negotiation. Polyamorous communities create supportive networks in which people can learn and practice these skills.

Those who had been isolated and then found organized polyamorous communities routinely commented on how much they learned about communication (among other things) from other polyamorists. Melody Lupine had initiated a polyamorous triad in her small Midwestern town where the threesome was secluded from other polyamorists:

> And unfortunately we didn't have any pool to communicate or no support groups back then. We lived in Ohio and it was the Midwest and again this wasn't heard of, there were no people around us, any of our close friends that we approached with it had a lot of judgments about it, and actually we got ostracized from several communities because of it . . . And again we didn't have very much support and didn't know—we ended up doing a lot of hurtful things to each other, and we didn't even realize. We just didn't have the communication tools and wasn't attentive of the other's needs, and we just didn't know how to make it work and how to do it.

Melody viewed role models who had previously navigated complexities, knew "how to make it work," and could show others "how to do it" as central to the successful function of her polyamorous family and individual emotional health.

Communication is key, not only in dealing with the emotional complexities of polyamorous relationships but also in negotiating boundaries structuring those multiplistic relationships.[54] While there are plenty of role models for people in monogamous relationships, they are fairly scarce for polyamorists, who create templates for their own relationships. Negotiating safer-sex agreements, boundaries structuring relationships with a variety of partners, and even the domestic division of labor among multiple partners and coparents requires extensive communication skills.

Poly relationships with poor communication tend to self-destruct rather rapidly. Morgan Majek said of the disastrous and short-lived relationship her husband, Carl, had with his first girlfriend, Janice: "They had both been expressing [to others] how hard it was to be with one another. They don't communicate; they don't talk to each other. So it just wasn't a match." Although Janice and Carl tried to communicate and had an intense sexual connection, their relationship did not last because of the incompatibility in their communication styles. Communication is so important in polyamorous relationships that, when it fails, the malfunction often overshadows other aspects of the relationship. Even the strongest sexual connection might not be enough to keep a poly relationship together if miscommunication spoils the emotional connection.

Polys use communication to get to know each other, and they often use *relationship maps* as a form of communication/foreplay possibly unique to polyamorous communities. Relationship maps are diagrams polys draw to explain their complex webs of relationships, generally with current and past lovers, the characteristics of the relationships (primary, secondary, fluid bonded, etc.), and lovers' lovers, when known. Vance, a twenty-seven-year-old white computer analyst, re-marked:

> Every first-time date includes a map of everyone I am seeing at the time, relevant past relationships, and as much of their [his lovers'] sexual history as I can muster. Inevitably I find areas where my lovers overlap with the new person. It helps us figure out where we are and talk about [sexually transmitted] diseases.

Usually everyone involved in the courting episode draws their own map, and these discussions almost inevitably lead to disclosing the presence of any sexually transmitted infections.

OVERLAP WITH OTHER COMMUNITIES

There is considerable overlap between polyamorous communities and other subcultures including geeks, gamers, and science fiction fans, people with unconventional political or spiritual views, and other sexual minorities such as kinksters, bisexuals, swingers, and gays and lesbians. Some polys endorse the overlap as a paradigm shift that enclosed all forms of alternative relationships. A woman writing online, who identified herself as "Mary," stated:

> I'm very interested in all new paradigms of relationship and sex, be they poly, Tantra, Buddhism, etc. It seems to me that they share common philosophies of negotiation, trust, honesty and ethics; as opposed to the cast-iron "morality" of traditional marriage. I'm a queer friendly straight girl writer/performer and PhD student, living

in Australia with my longtime bf [boy friend]. I'm not actively poly—
I'm one of those people who finds just one primary relationship a
pretty major thing to deal with, both emotionally and physically. (My
SO [significant other] and I are open to the potential of the occasional friendly/loving fuck-buddy fling—just not multiple "intense" relationships.)

While "Mary" did not wish to expand beyond the one primary relationship that she found a "pretty major thing to deal with," she nonetheless cast herself, and was welcomed by online community members, as
an ally to polyamorous people and those involved in what she viewed as
natural affiliates. Polyamorous communities frequently welcome allies
and do not require them to engage in multiple-partner relationships in
order to be accepted into the sexually permissive environment that
supports those who question a variety of cultural norms.

Unconventional People

Polyamory appears to be especially appealing to geeks, gamers, science
fiction fans, and people with unconventional religious or philosophical
views. Once someone has stepped outside the mainstream, it is easier to
continue considering alternatives. Usually people who become polyamorous have already done other unconventional things or held unconventional ideas: Polyamory is not usually the first step "outside of the box."

While many people play online or board games, not all are *gamers*:
Gamers are a special breed that take their play very seriously. One
version of the gamer is the LARPer, or Live Action Role Player, who
dresses in costume and plays a game in person, physically present with
the other players in a designated space. Organizations such as the Society for Creative Anachronism (SCA) provide LARPers with opportunities to play with others in costume and battle regalia.

Science fiction fans who read or watch media that portrays alternative visions of the future are also well represented among poly communities. Heinlein's work, especially *Stranger in a Strange Land*,[55] is probably the most influential body of science fiction in the polyamorous
community. *Stranger*, as many polys affectionately refer to the novel,
relates the story of a human man raised on Mars who returns to Earth
and founds a new religion that includes nonmonogamous relationships.

Rimmer's work, particularly *The Harrad Experiment*,[56] set on a college campus that advocated sexual sharing and nonsexual nudity among students, is similarly influential in the formation and ideas of the polyamorous community. Both novels portray groups of people living together (mostly harmoniously) and sharing sexual partners. Many polys say that they read one or both books at a time in their lives when they had not previously considered multiple-partner relationships, and they ended up using the novels as models for how to build their own expanded intimate networks.

In addition to the geeks and scifi fans, there are other people with unconventional views among the ranks of the polyamorous. Anarchists often favor nonmonogamy because of the implicit freedom of choice, and Pagans who worship multiple god/esses have a spiritual orientation that embraces multiplicity. Such strange compatriots as libertarians, feminists, and Unitarian Universalists all value polyamory for the equal/gender-neutral opportunity it provides.

Kinksters

One of the primary overlapping communities is comprised of people who practice BD (bondage and discipline), Ds (dominance and submission), or SM (sadism and masochism), otherwise known as BDSM or more generally kinky sex. There are a number of similarities between the polyamorous and BDSM subcultures. Both are composed of members willing to challenge social norms structuring "vanilla" (the BDSM term for traditional sex) or monogamous relationships. Negotiation is centrally important to both communities, necessary to both structure relationships and to create agreements supporting the relationships. Some polyamorists practice BDSM to varying degrees, and many kinksters (people who engage in kinky sex) have multiple partners with whom they "play" or "scene." For kinksters, "playing" means engaging in episodes that involved explicitly sexual acts (up to and including penetration), or simply have a sexual tone but did not involve what others might consider sex per se. A "scene" is a sexual encounter negotiated around a specific script with detailed discussion of what will or will not happen and a "safe word" that immediately stops the scene if the submissive finds the stimulation or interaction too intense.[57]

Bisexuals

The popularity of bisexuality among polys encourages close connections with bisexual organizations and communities. Some polys discover polyamory through their involvement in bisexual politics or organizations, and the overlapping members and politics the poly and bisexual communities share are so extensive that some people like Earl, a white man at a dinner party, think that "bisexuality and polyamory are two sides of the same coin."

Swingers

Polys also share many practices and attitudes with swingers, and some community members as well. Like polys, swingers are predominantly white,[58] educated,[59] middle and upper-middle class people with professional or managerial employment.[60] Both groups appear to be gaining members through Internet contact.[61] Swingers and some polys distinguish between their primary partners (usually a spouse or spouselike relationship) and other sexual partners. Swingers have a code of etiquette focused on ethical treatment of spouses rather than moral guidelines, very much like poly folks.[62] Both polyamorists and swingers use honesty to normalize nonconformist sexual behavior, stigmatize people in "monogamous" relationships who cheat, talk a lot about how to manage jealousy, and each sees their common focus on truthful communication as leading to healthier relationships and better sex.[63]

Henshel argued that, because the men in her sample initiated swinging 68 percent of the time, males were the dominant force in the swinging situation.[64] I would add that swingers' focus on female bisexuality as entertaining for men and far more acceptable than the virtually prohibited male bisexuality exposes the underlying sexism and homophobia in both swing and poly communities. They even share a mascot: the Bonobo chimpanzee, whose interactions in the wild tend toward cooperation and group sex.[65]

There are, however, important differences between swingers and polyamorists. Swingers have no practice of group marriage, and the female/male couple is clearly the basic unit in swing settings. Swingers tend to be more heterosexual and far more politically conservative than polyamorists.[66] Swingers tend to live as couples, often married, and so can often pass for conventional monogamists far more easily than poly-amorists with multiple spice who live or attend public functions togeth-er.

In contrast to those poly people who see their polyamorousness as an innate orientation, swingers often characterize their multiple-partner sexual practices as purely a lifestyle choice. Gould draws a distinction between recreational swingers (which he reports dominate "the Life-style") and utopian swingers, by far the minority. He and others in swinging settings cast the latter as more revolutionary in that utopian swingers want to change the norms relating to marriage; the recreation-al swingers have no such intent.[67] Polyamorists, with their desire for social change, are far more closely aligned with the minority utopian swingers.

These last two differences—viewing desire for multiple partners as innate or as a choice, and a desire or lack thereof to change traditional familial and gender roles—are the most important differences with polyamorists. Swingers' focus on choice and ability to pass make them a less cohesive group, more of a collection of individuals who share a common interest in their personal sexual satisfaction rather than social change. Polys' emphasis on innate characteristics, desire for social change, and the popularity of platonic socializing far more extensively than swingers makes polyamorists members of a community and move-ment. As a result, polys have more philosophical overlap with gays and lesbians, who share these crucial traits as both a movement and a com-munity, rather than swingers.

Lesbians and Gays

While polyamorous communities have tremendous overlaps with some sexual minorities, they also lack a significant intersection with others that initially appear to be natural affiliates. Polyamorists mirror gays and lesbians in many areas, including bearing the brunt of social stigma, the risk of losing child custody, difficulty finding partners in the general populace, and making decisions about when to come out and to whom. Even with all of these similarities, there is a glaring absence of lesbians and gay men in the mainstream polyamorous subculture. There are several potential reasons for this.

A lack of lesbians in polyamorous communities could be due to lesbian discomfort with bisexual women. Tina, a thirty-six-year-old white urban planner, reflected:

> I identified as a lesbian for so long, and I really enjoyed women's energy, just getting together and talking about things. When I actually got into the poly women's group I thought that most of them would be lesbians, and I was very surprised to find a majority of them are heterosexual or bi with a male primary partner, and I was like, that's kind of different . . . I guess I've always identified as bisexual, but I called myself lesbian for many years so I could feel more comfortable hanging out in the lesbian community. There's a lot of politics around that.

Lesbians who view bisexual women with contempt are unlikely to be comfortable in a setting so heavily populated with bisexual women, especially when the bisexual women are so highly valued in poly communities. Indeed, Rust found that the lesbians in her study held decidedly negative views against bisexual women as "sexual opportunists, fickle lovers, traitors, political cowards, or fence-sitters."[68]

Alternately, lesbians may not wish to subject themselves to male sexual advances, and the comparative dearth of available women in some poly communities could contribute to what one woman attending a community potluck termed a "feeding frenzy," when men "swarm like sharks around women who seem available." Finally, lesbians may not wish to compete with men for the potentially rare available woman who is seeking additional partners. These factors could combine to encourage lesbians to date within their own poly circles rather than brave the masculinity in mainstream poly communities.

Gay men might feel no need for additional support for multiple-partner practices. Though some gay men have a well-documented habit of establishing multiple-partner relationships,[69] most do not identify themselves as polyamorous. I observed an almost complete absence of gay men in the polyamorous communities of both the Midwest and the California Bay Area. Gay and lesbian communities in the Midwest are smaller and less developed, but the Bay Area hosts one of the largest and most well-organized gay and lesbian communities in the United States. This obvious lack of gays and lesbians in Bay Area poly communities, compared to the large representation of bisexuals, is especially noteworthy. It is possible that nonmonogamy is so thoroughly accepted in gay male culture that most gay men feel no need for additional support from polyamorous communities. Further, it is likely that gay men in multiple-partner relationships have no desire to confront the possibility of homophobia in many polyamorous communities.

Javier, a thirty-five-year-old Mexican American man, and Christian, a thirty-nine-year-old white man, attended a national polyamory conference in California in order to reach out to the polyamorous community. They had been engaged in a successful nonmonogamous relationship for five years and wished to meet others with similar interests. Christian commented:

> Not many [men] we know identify as polyamorous but over 90 percent are what I would term "poly sexually oriented," meaning they have multiple sexual partners outside of their primary relationships or date a lot or "hook up" a lot. Many are polysexual at least. I know of very few, if any, monogamous male-male relationships, though I do know of many female-female monogamous relationships. We do not know many polyamorous gay men . . . In the male-male sex world there is on the one hand a wish to lifelong monogamy and the picket fence partnership. But reality is most male-male relationships have outside sexual encounters that run the range from shared encounters with the two partners to complete secondary, one-on-one relationships.

Their perceived isolation as polyamorous men in a gay world drew Javier and Christian to attend the national polyamorous conference. At the conference, however, both men said they felt very awkward with the primarily white, heterosexual, and bisexual crowd. While their mutual bisexuality offered some potential point of overlap with the other conference attendees, they nonetheless felt marginalized. "You just don't see folks like us around here much." Not only was there an absence of other male couples, there were hardly any people of color. As a mixed race Latino and white couple, they felt very out of place and told me they would probably not attend another poly conference.

Thaddeus, a thirty-five-year-old white musician who identified as queer, spent most of his time in what he termed the "gay subculture." He did not, however, identify this gay subculture as a community, as he did with polyamorous communities:

[Midwestern town] is the first place I've found that has any sort of interactive polyamorous community and is something that I would call a community because they know each other. If somebody's car broke down they could call somebody else for help. The same cannot be said of what we call the gay community, which I continue to insist is not a community but a subculture. In some places there's community . . . these are places that have a very high concentration of gay people living there on a permanent basis and because they do know each other it does tend to form community, but in general, no. If you walked down the street and were hit by a car you can't count on help from somebody just because you're gay. And that's unfortunate.

Thaddeus saw more differences between gay subcultures and polyamorous communities than the lack of coherent social norms and willingness to assist each other. He also observed a profound difference in the way each group handled multiple-partner relationships:

They [most polyamorous people] don't think of gay men as being polyamorous because we are so free sexually anyway. It's part of our subculture. What isn't part of our subculture is emotional relationships in multiple terms. Sexual relationships? Sure! That's all over the place, but emotional relationships, it's rare. You find occasional triads, you find occasional vees, one-timers or secondaries or one person with two lovers that may or may not interact. But those folks still don't think of themselves as polyamorous, they're still just calling themselves gay. Because in that subculture, pretty much, your style is your style and nobody's gonna cram monogamy down your throat there.

Thaddeus felt that he was different from most people in mainstream gay subcultures because he wanted so much emotional connection that he doubted one lover could ever fill what he saw as his vast emotional needs. While he said his high sex drive was one of the reasons he wanted to have poly relationships, the more important factor was "emotional engagement, clearly . . . I've never been satisfied with relationships that were simply sexually based."

Still, some polyamorists view gays and lesbians as natural affiliates and even patterned themselves after gay and lesbian activists. Mim Chapman, a member of the activist-oriented group in New York, wrote on the web:

> GLBT's and their allies are fighting to give male and male/female and female couples the right to enter the ark of social acceptance. Polyamorists are now taking on the second half of the Noah syndrome, the two by two bit.[70]

Gay and lesbian people have been organizing politically for more than thirty years, and while some polyamorists try to learn from the success of that identity-based movement, obstacles remain that keep polyamory from being as politically potent as the LGBT movement. For one thing, polys do not always identify themselves as a political movement, preferring to focus instead on their own emotional well-being and developing tools to navigate multiple relationships. Another reason polys are less politicized is that polyamory is such a fluid relationship style, and community members disagree about who counts as poly and why, that it is difficult to use as a base for identity politics.

Finally, although exclusively same-sex (nonbisexual) relationships are rare in most mainstream poly communities, there are lesbian polyamorous subcultures in some large cities in the United States, such as Seattle and the California Bay Area. Unfortunately, none of them volunteered to participate in the research, so they do not appear in this book. Books such as Celeste West's *Lesbian Polyfidelity* and Marcia Munsun and Judith Stelboum's *The Lesbian Polyamory Reader* also indicate the existence of lesbian polyamorists.

POLY FATIGUE

While poly people get many benefits from their relationships and association with other poly community members, sometimes they get tired of the drama and constant negotiation. Norman, a thirty-year-old writer, decided he was done with polyamorous relationships because

> I just can't handle this shit anymore! I mean, there are marriages that last for forty years that don't have the amount of drama you can squeeze into a four-month poly relationship. I mean, dramatic to the point of being toxic! Still, I think I will stick around the poly community [as a monogamous person] because I have found kindred souls here. There is a fellowship core of poly people that feels really good to me.

Norman, and others like him who had decided to return to a monogamous relationship style, often continued to feel accepted in the polyamorous community and chose to remain associated for social and political
reasons.

Others were far more disappointed with polyamorous community
interaction. After twenty-five years of polyamorous relationships, the
community had not lived up to Emmanuella's expectations:

> I wanted everybody to grow the hell up and start acting like it mat-
> tered and get past the petty jealousies and talk about why it was
> important to open up relationships, why monogamy is such a hard-
> ship for both men and women, why the nuclear family is so damaging
> to children, why communal living, whether it's physically, in terms of
> proximity, or in terms of support, is so important. I thought those
> things would have occurred by now and in some faraway places ran-
> domly it is occurring somewhat, I'm told, but each one under its own
> principles, and polyamory is a very loose term for what most people
> assume are very loose people. And that is not the thing I want to be
> associated with. I wanted it to be the answer to nonmonogamy. I
> thought that it would be making more sense by now and it would be
> something I would be proud to introduce my children, to share with
> them, to say this is it. And instead my son says you're a bunch of
> aging hippies. I want it to be more than that, to radicalize the con-
> cept and to make it more inclusive of gays and lesbians.

Emmanuella was disillusioned by what she saw as the ultimate fate of
polyamorous community politics. Rather than revolutionizing marriage,
family, and relationships, she thought the polyamorous movement had
squandered its potential on bickering among "a bunch of aging hippies."

Some long-term polyamorists are more optimistic, still hopeful of
impacting real social change. Still others are so upset with the community and their relationships within it that they stop identifying as polyamorists and either become monogamous or begin identifying simply as
"nonmonogamous." Most of them are not represented in this book.

4

ISSUES FACING POLY RELATIONSHIPS

MY STORY

"I realize that I'm in love with Steve," I said, looking at Rick with my heart pounding and a terrible tightness in my chest. His eyes clenched in pain and he said, "I really did not want to do this tonight. I got your mom to stay with the kids tomorrow so we could talk, and I already told you that I really didn't want to process tonight before that conversation. I don't want you to be with Steve, it's not working. In fact, I think we should get married and be monogamous." In that moment I felt something break and knew that I would never really love Rick again. If we had not had children I would have gone right home and started packing because I was out of there. It scared me to death, and I buried it as soon as I realized it, spending the next five years trying to pretend it hadn't happened and searching for some way I could save my relationship with Rick. But we had been through too much, for too long, for him to suddenly shift from polyamory to marital monogamy.

✿ ✿ ✿ ✿ ✿

During the fifteen years I have studied polyamory, my role as a researcher has gone from civilian (no research intent but a desire to find out about it for my own purposes), to peripheral (deciding to research the topic and "coming out" to the community as a researcher), and then complete member (having a polyamorous relationship myself) before returning once again to a peripheral role.[1] That path is actually quite common to poly relationships, in that they tend to be fluid, flexible, and changing. Relatively few of those I spoke with kept their relationships in the precise form that they were when I initially interviewed them. More often, they retained connection and continuity with the same people in their lives, but the form or specific expression of the relationship would shift over time.

Quite importantly, this fluidity in these relationships did not necessarily translate to high levels of partner attrition. Rather than cycling through and discarding a parade of partners, most respondents retained contact with significant others over long periods of time, but the form that contact took often shifted over the years. For example, in my own life this has taken the form of a twenty-three-year (to date) relationship with Rick, the father of my children. For the first fifteen years we were "together" as a couple, and for the last eight years as coparents and sometimes friends. We still know each other and communicate regularly. We remain fixtures in each other's lives—available to consult, collaborate, help, or argue—though the form of our relationship has changed over time.

THE BEGINNING

I was a twenty-three-year-old undergraduate student when I met Rick in 1993 at a university in Northern California. While I had been in love once before, I had very little dating or sexual experience, so I was not ready for it when I fell in love with Rick so quickly. On our first date Rick told me that he never wanted to get married or be monogamous. I thought, "Whatever, freak, you are not going to last long anyway," and said, "OK, I guess." Rick elaborated on his fantasy family with two women who loved each other and him, and how it might look like a harem but we would really be challenging patriarchal notions of marriage and monogamy with our harmonious, triadic union. My original casual attitude shifted, and as our relationship became more serious I got increasingly uncomfortable with Rick's desire for nonmonogamy.

Unicorn Hunting and Couple Privilege

Though we didn't know it, Rick's ideal family fit the poly stereotype of female-male couples approaching the poly community to find a wife so closely that I came to think of it later as Unicorn Hunter's Syndrome. The plethora of personal ads from unicorn hunters on poly websites and the ubiquitous presence of couples cruising at poly social events hoping to meet available women make it abundantly clear that the stereotype is well grounded in reality. As my relationship with Rick deepened, he elaborated on his ideal triad in which we would find a woman we both loved equally and the three of us would live together in expanded bliss, raising children and making each other happy. Implicit in his discussion was the unexamined assumption that whatever woman we bonded with would not have other partners already but would join us in our lives without any attendant relationships of her own. Such a myopic view of a woman willing to fold herself into someone else's existing plan as if she were a mere ingredient can only exist if that fantasized woman is (at best) two-dimensional—certainly not a multidimensional human with plans and lovers of her own. Polyamorists term this dynamic *couple privilege*—a narrow focus on the couple's needs and desires as the primary or sole determinant of a relationship at the possible expense of the unicorn's feelings, desires, or even full personhood.

Over time, the ongoing discussion with Rick expanded to include other aspects of what unicorn hunter couples often desire—a woman willing to join in the domestic life of the household, helping with cooking, cleaning, and child care. When it became clear that Rick wanted a large family and I was open to having children but also wanted an academic career, we imagined finding a female partner who might want to bear or adopt (and care for) more children. Envisioning our mythical girlfriend in a domestic role while one or both of us worked for pay was yet another symptom of a unicorn hunter couple: basically we were looking for a wife with an unconscious arrogance reminiscent of male privilege in more conventional relationships. In polyamorous lingo, we were seeking the hot bi babe.

Hot Bi Babes

The arrangement of triadic sex between one man and two women was the most popular relationship form sought by the polyamorous men who attended support groups, frequented online chat rooms and discussion boards, and wrote personal ads in polyamorous online or print publications. Most polyamorous men did not have regular access to simultaneous sex with multiple women. Enough of them were able to occasionally fulfill that fantasy, however, to keep the hope of its occurrence alive for the others. This common fantasy seemed to appeal to a large number of polyamorous men, and it served as one of the most distinguishing features of hegemonic hypermasculinity among polyamorous men.[2]

Some polyamorous men were successful in living out the seemingly pervasive heterosexual male fantasy of having sex simultaneously with multiple women, the proverbial "girl-on-girl" scene depicted so frequently in pornography produced for heterosexual men. These men established triadic sexual relationships with two women or had sexual encounters with bisexual women and were occasionally joined by the women's female lovers. Ironically, some men found simultaneous sex with two women to be "not all that." In their fantasies, the men were the center of attention and the women related to each other and him simultaneously. In reality, however, some men reported that the women were more focused on each other and less interested in the man than he would have liked.

For example, Max Amore reported that he was less entertained by the triadic sexual encounters he had with his then-wife, Louise, and their girlfriend, Monique Mayfield.

> I guess things lasted for about five or six months with us getting together regularly. She [Monique] would come over with her kids and we would all have dinner together, watch a movie or play a game, something like that. Then the kids would take over the downstairs and the adults would go upstairs. Pretty quickly I got bored with it, but Louise and Monique were infatuated with each other and I felt like I should go along for the ride. But yeah, being with the two of them didn't turn out to be all that for me, though I think they really liked being with each other. The kids all got along great and Louise and Monique were really happy with the arrangement for a while, but it never worked out to what I really wanted it to be.
>
> It wasn't that long of a haul, less than a year. I just felt, I dunno, less attention than I wanted, less of a focus with three people than you have when it's only the two of you in the bed. Not like they [Louise and Monique] were jerks to me or anything, I just didn't, I wasn't feeling it.

Even though Louise and Max were able to establish a relationship with a bisexual woman, their triadic sexual and personal encounters left Max unsatisfied and wanting more attention.

Some men who entered a polyamorous community seeking a triad with two women changed their focus once it became clear that such a relationship was extremely difficult to find. Mark and Evelyn Coach had originally sought the HBB relationship, to no avail:

> When we started this we were sort of invested in the idea of finding the mythical hot bi babe who would come and join our relationship and what happened instead was the first person that she [Evelyn] got involved with, this lover in Seattle that she'd been involved with before who certainly—he didn't fit the hot bi babe category as we had discussed it, so at this point while we sort of had this vision of the larger family, we are no longer attached to any particular geometry of how it will occur.

Mark and Evelyn altered their expectations when it appeared their HBB was unlikely to materialize. Many polyamorists related similar stories of their unsuccessful quests for a HBB and the varied impacts that had had on their relationships. Some retained their original goal of seeking her out and looked for fifteen or more years, to no avail. Others found her, only to discover the relationship did not meet their expectations. I spoke with very few who had engaged in a lasting relationship with a HBB as she is popularly conceived, though I found far more polyaffective triads with one woman and two men.

I propose three potential explanations for this HBB phenomenon. The greater social acceptance of sex between women, stigma of bisexual men, and the scarcity of available female partners might combine to create a setting in which bisexual women become fetish objects. Much like monogamous society and swinging subcultures,[3] sex between women was more socially acceptable within polyamorous communities than was sex between men. The HBB was implicitly a woman—and not the woman already engaged in the female/male couple, but the free agent, who would be added to create the triadic sexual encounter. Sex among women, especially if there was potential for a man to "get in on it," was entertaining for most polyamorous (and many monogamous) men.

Men who engaged in sex with men, on the other hand, raised the specter of homophobia. Men interested in "getting in on" group sex with other men must have same-sex attraction—thus undermining their hegemonic heterosexual identity. Valorization of bisexual women and the stigma of bisexual men paralleled standards in general society where many heterosexual men enjoy female bisexuality more than male bisexuality.

While polyamorous people did not expressly state that men were not the focus of the HBB fantasy, it was obvious in their conversations. People either spoke explicitly of seeking women or used female pronouns in their friendly banter about desirable partners. At one party I attended, I stood in the kitchen with a group of six or seven polyamorists who were discussing their lovers. A white man in his late forties made a joke about the perfect lover everyone sought but could not seem to find. He ended with, "But she would knock all of your socks off, no doubt!" His story portrayed an idealized version of *everyone's* elusive lover, who was a woman. The group included men and women, so a desire to have sex for all of us indicated that the idealized woman would be bisexual.

Some bisexual men, on the other hand, reported feeling constrained by potential social disapproval when considering disclosure of their sexual orientation. Sven Heartland had sought a bisexual man for seven years with whom he and Shelly could form a triad. Shelly and Sven Heartland, both white professionals with office jobs, each have a daughter from a previous marriage (Elise and Kimber), and also have a daughter together (Alice). Sven's first marriage ended in a bitter divorce when his now ex-wife discovered he was having clandestine sex with men. In an effort to avoid repeating the mistakes of his first marriage, Sven was honest with Shelly about his bisexuality from the beginning of their relationship, though he remained cautious of identifying himself as bisexual to new members of his polyamorous community:

> When I meet someone new in the community or a new person attends the support group meeting I am always careful what I say at first until I can see what they are like. I don't want a negative reaction, so I use pronouns like "they" and "we" instead of saying "he" when I am talking about me and Shelly and Adam, just in case.

The majority of bisexual women in the polyamorous community did not share Sven's caution. The women, far from concealing their sexual orientation, enjoyed the highest social status in the community. This relationship between gender and bisexuality indicated homophobia against men with which women did not have to contend.

Another possible reason for the valorization of bisexual women and the stigma of bisexual men was the scarcity of available or "free-floating" female partners. Many polyamorous women were already partnered with numerous people, and single or available women were rare at community gatherings. Single or available men seemed abundant and more willing to entertain casual sexual relationships. Scarcity would increase women's value in relationships, bisexual or not.[4]

Ironically, some elements of the polyamorous community reversed the HBB scenario, and sexualized bisexual men more so than women. Thaddeus, a thirty-five-year-old white musician who identified as queer, commented:

> I've certainly not encountered a lot of homophobia [in polyamorous communities]. I'm sure, mind you, that most of the men that I've met identify as polyamorous, um, wouldn't consider a male partner, I do know a couple that identify as bisexual, um, I know one of those who has ads in the [poly personal ads website], but you know, "I've never had a relationship with a man." They're polyamorous but they'll pursue women for relationships and men just for sex.

Clearly, some polyamorists viewed men, and not just bisexual women, as sexual objects. Joya Solarity's emphatic statement emphasized Thaddeus's assertion: "I have really intensely been attracted to bi boys; extremely, intensely attracted to bi boys . . . I just can't get enough of bi boys." Even with this intense attraction for bisexual "boys," she reported:

> And inside of that, I'm finding my attention is again drawn more toward women than before. And I feel like my connections there mean more to me and I'm finding that I want to play more with boys, just kind of play, a casual thing.

Although Joya refrained from stigmatizing bisexual men, and indeed intentionally sought their company, her relationships with them were primarily sexual in nature. Joya reserved her intense emotional connections for relationships with women.

Polyamorous ambivalence regarding male bisexuality and homosexuality was a point of contention among community members. Some in the San Francisco Bay Area, renowned for its acceptance of same-sex relationships and home of a decidedly sex-positive polyamorous community, appeared to have greater acceptance of bisexual men. While in the South Bay, I attended a "bisexual coffee night" in a local coffee shop. There was jovial conversation and flirting, and at one point, two men sitting on a couch at one corner of the circle of attendees began kissing passionately. Conversation died out as we all sat watching the men kiss. Slowly the men became aware of the silence around them and broke their embrace, followed rapidly by cheering and applause from their impromptu audience members. Clearly, the group had appreciated the erotic moment. Even in the Bay Area, however, bisexual men were not as highly valorized as were bisexual women.

Some of the men in my sample discussed their awareness of differing community standards regarding bisexual men and women and the apparent homophobia it revealed. Acknowledging the double standard, many still opined that polyamorists were far less homophobic and more tolerant of men who engaged in a wide variety of nonhegemonic activities than was the general society. Norman, a thirty-year-old African American writer, explained that polyamorous men tended to be more open-minded than monogamous men, especially when it came to men having sex with men.

> Polyamorous men are more comfortable with bi and homosexual men than straight men usually are. Even if you don't wanna have a man touch your ass, you're still cool with the fact that they like to touch other men's asses.

Nonetheless, Norman mentioned a double standard that glorified sex between women far more so than sex between men, as long as the sex between women was "entertaining" to men. His perception of lesser degrees of homophobia in polyamorous settings was inflected by his simultaneous awareness of the objectification of bisexual women. The relationship between gender and bisexuality within the polyamorous community was as complex as the relationship between polyamorous men and masculinity. Both women and men could be sexualized as sex toys, though it was far more common for women among the communities I studied. Bisexuality was an asset for polyamorous women, but fewer men viewed it as such. Some bisexual polyamorous men even reported fearing it might be a disadvantage.

CIVILIAN RESEARCH ROLE

During my second semester of graduate school I heard a National Public Radio interview with Ryam Nearing, who published *Loving More* magazine at the time. She explained that the magazine was for people in openly conducted nonmonogamous relationships—something she called *polyamory*. My subsequent Internet search revealed that the *Loving More* editors were based nearby and that they hosted community meetings and support groups. Rick and I began attending events such as a public discussion forum at a local library, a local support group where I could ask questions and express my fears about polyamorous relationships, and social events such as movie nights or group hikes. Many of the people profiled and mentioned in this book were people I met there.

Marriage?

Deeply in love and looking for some definition to our relationship, when I was twenty-seven I asked Rick to marry me. He declined, reminding me that he had been clear from the beginning about his disdain for marriage as a patriarchal institution designed to give men ownership over women and the ability to hand property down to male children the men are certain that they fathered. I countered that marriage could be anything we made it, and we went around that topic for two years with no resolution. Finally Rick said that he would marry me if, in place of where the groom would usually say vows, he could turn and tell the people in attendance, "I don't want to be doing this. Marriage is a sham, and Elisabeth is forcing me to do this." Unsurprisingly, I declined. In a move I interpreted as caving in, I agreed to remain together unmarried and dropped the issue. Soon after we started trying to have a child, and ten months later our son was born.

PERIPHERAL RESEARCH ROLE

The more time I spent with the polyamorists, the more I liked them, and the more interested I became in them from a sociological standpoint. About a year and a half after my introduction to the local polyamorous community, I chose to do a study on a local poly community for my term paper in a graduate course. As part of my study, I became increasingly close with several local polyamorists, whom I found like-minded and friendly. At this point, I began to regularly attend the local monthly support group for polyamorous women.

I had forged close friendships with several women in the setting prior to considering it as a research area, and these relationships continued as I transitioned to a research role. The transition itself was sometimes challenging: occasionally I felt uncomfortable in groups, knowing that I would take notes on the interactions and that some group members might have been unaware of my status as a researcher. Fox felt similar discomfort when she felt compelled to "tread a line between overt and covert roles" in her investigation of a punk social scene.[5] Although I enjoyed socializing with polyamorists, I remained "acutely aware of differences between members and [myself]" and thus retained a peripheral membership role.[6]

Communication, Honesty, and Sabotage

The most important poly relationship tool is honest communication. Authors, community members, and bloggers—everyone repeats the "poly mantra" of "communicate, communicate, communicate." Polyamorists agree that honesty and communication are essential to successful poly relationships because they are prerequisites for trust, and without trust polyamory will not work because people in the relationships will not feel safe or confident in their partners' abilities and willingness to be forthright.

Communication is not simply volume of contact but also techniques of how to communicate effectively. Poly folks often attempt to incorporate radical honesty and nonviolent communication in their relationship, with the outcome of using *I* statements as opposed to *you* or accusatory statements and listening carefully, which often means repeating back what they think the other person is saying and taking a break to cool off before reengaging if a conversation gets too heated.

In my case, the volume of communication Rick and I had obscured the fact that we were not being clear with each other. While I was well aware of my reluctance to be polyamorous and my attempts to manipulate our relationship to retain a monogamous tenor, I was not aware of it consciously at the time of how tenuous I felt Rick's connection to be and thus failed to communicate that to him. Part of that was lack of clarity on my part, and part of it was fear of his response if he perceived me to be giving him an ultimatum about being monogamous with me.

This ongoing exposure to the polys' ideas and novel forms of relationship had an impact on my relationship with Rick, and socializing regularly with polyamorists spurred many conversations between the two of us. We embarked upon a slow process of opening our relationship to outside partners and, in so doing, made a number of mistakes common to "newbies" or those who are first attempting polyamory. For instance, we decided to try a "don't ask, don't tell" (DADT) version of a relationship we had heard about from others attending polyamorous functions. Popular among newbies and swingers, long-term polyamorists generally eschew DADT relationships as doomed to fail in weirdness and unintentional deceit. As was characteristic of that type of relationship, Rick and I decided that we could each have outside lovers as long as the other person didn't have to hear about it. To that polyamorous standard, we added an additional rule that we could only see others while traveling separately, and these "road" relationships were never to interfere with the home relationship.

I saw this last rule as virtually prohibiting outside relationships, because we rarely traveled at all and, when we did, we did so as a family. The agreement, in my eyes, was a win-win situation. Rick could think of himself as a polyamorous person and revel in the freedom of the possibility, however remote, that he could have another lover. I, on the other hand, had no intention of finding us a girlfriend, and I could not readily imagine the circumstances in which Rick would do so, either. Reluctant to have a poly relationship but worn down by the constant conversation, I manipulated an impossible agreement to sabotage any hope of a poly relationship becoming real.

Such manipulation is also a common newbie mistake. All too often, couples with unresolved power issues or poor communication begin to seek a poly relationship even though one of the members does not actually wish to be polyamorous. In some cases, one partner wants to have access to multiple lovers himself or herself but is not actually comfortable with her or his partner having sex with others and so creates various impediments to that partner being able to establish additional relationships. These impediments can take the form of recurrent crises that require immediate attention each time the partner has a date scheduled and prohibit the date from actually happening. In other cases, a partner will object to each potential partner for a variety of reasons that may or may not appear to be reasonable at the time but culminate in the reality that none of the people the partner wishes to date are acceptable to the saboteur. In my case, I negotiated rules that appeared reasonable on the surface but effectively foreclosed any possibility that either Rick or I would actually be able to initiate a tryst with anyone else. All of these scenarios share a common thread of manipulation and sabotage rather than direct and clear communication—common pitfalls that routinely ensnare inexperienced polyamorists. Over the course of this phase of our relationship, I accidentally became pregnant again and had our second child.

Rick and I continued to discuss our relationship and reached another stage in the gradual opening to additional partners. As I had anticipated, we had never used the "don't ask, don't tell" arrangement. Our new agreement allowed openly conducted, same-sex relationships in our home area. Again, I agreed because I thought it incredibly unlikely that such a relationship would ever come to exist. Rick had no interest in sex with other men, and I was not seeking other partners, so I did not see how it would realistically work out for us to see others. The idea was satisfying to him and nonthreatening to me, and it allowed us each to feel some degree of comfort as we sought to figure out how to live our lives together. Rick saw himself as a polyamorist, and I viewed myself as a monogamist in polyamorous clothing. Even as I developed close ties with local community members, I did not seriously consider multiple-partner relationships as a possibility for myself.

About this time, Rick's close friends Theresa and Jonathan visited from California. During the many conversations we had that long weekend, Rick and I spent some time discussing our quasi-polyamorous relationship with them, and Theresa called several weeks later to tell me she had a crush on me and wanted to see what developed. Theresa and I included Rick and Jonathan in several phone conversations. Rick was thrilled. He thought that a quad with close friends could be another form of the ideal alternative family he sought. Theresa was uncertain if she wished to rekindle the sexual relationship she had had with Rick years ago. Jonathan was similarly ambivalent about a sexual relationship between Rick and Theresa, though he said he was "fine" with a sexual relationship between Theresa and me. Jonathan thought he might be able to become attracted to me, though, and considered triadic sexual encounters with Theresa, him, and me a strong possibility. Characteristic of long-distance poly relationships, we spent a lot of time trying to get to know each other more with phone calls and emails as we considered what shape the relationship might take, given the fact that we lived almost two thousand miles apart.

Once again, Rick and I did not test our agreement by taking additional lovers. Our discussions, however, progressed, and we decided to finally completely open our relationship to other partners. In retrospect, our reasons seem clearer to us now than they did then. I had grown exceedingly tired of the conversation and the endless consideration. Rick remained hesitant to seek a lover himself and hoped that, if he just waited long enough, I would find us a woman. So we agreed to an arrangement that allowed us to seek a girlfriend in our local area, which neither one of us intended to implement (though we did not know that of each other at the time).

Entrée into Polyamory

During this period, I traveled to California in the hope of collecting data that were more varied from a more racially and ethnically diverse polyamorous community. While in California, I visited Theresa and Jonathan. The visit was awkward for me. I felt increasingly uncomfortable as Theresa expressed her amorous feelings for me verbally and physically. I admitted that I was not experiencing reciprocal feelings, and she retreated, feeling hurt and rejected. I left Jonathan and Theresa's house feeling confused, upset, and more convinced of my lack of desire for multiple partners. If I did not wish to explore a sexual relationship with these wonderful people whom I already loved as friends, I reasoned, there must be no one other than Rick who would spark my interest. I thought, after all, I must be monogamous. I enjoyed the interviews and had a great time socializing with community members, but once again I refrained from sexual interaction.

I called Rick at home and explained my lack of desire for Theresa and all the other suitors in California and across the years. At that point we had been discussing our potential poly relationship several times a week for almost ten years, and I had long since wearied of the conversation. I told him that I was probably never going to be actively polyamorous myself, but I would consider a poly/mono relationship in which he would be polyamorous and I would remain monogamous. After even more discussion, he created an online profile and began attempting to date.

While Rick and I moved with glacial slowness toward polyamory and discussed every aspect of it in excruciating detail, others rush in, and still others evolve into the relationship. In chapter 2 I discussed different ways of thinking about and being polyamorous, and my findings are that those with a polyamorous sexual/relational orientation frequently established open relationships in their youths and came to identify as poly later. More often, people would have monogamous relationships first and then become polyamorous either by a purposeful decision or through happenstance. Because Rick and I exemplify an extreme example of purposeful decision and I discuss that in such length throughout the chapter, here I focus on relationships formed via happenstance.

The most successful poly relationships that begin with happenstance usually include people exploring the possibility to mutually open the relationship prior to anyone acting as if she or he was in an open relationship. People who begin acting as if they are in open relationships and then try to negotiate their boundaries in retrospect—have affairs first and then confess or get caught and then try to discuss opening their relationships—often have disastrous results. Because honesty is crucial to the successful function of poly relationships, they often implode when founded on dishonesty. In the case of polyamory, it is generally much better to ask for permission first than forgiveness afterward.

There are some significant exceptions to this rule among my respondents. The Bayside triad with Cal, John, and Sara began with an affair between Sara, legally married to Cal, and John, in the process of divorcing someone else. Sara reported that her affair with John had been going on for barely a month, and she knew Cal was going to find out about it because he did the bills, and there was this new number all over my cell phone bill with like, hours of conversations in the middle of the night. So of course he was going to figure it out, how could he not? I was kind of deer-in-the-headlights, frozen waiting for the disaster to start, and it never came.

Cal: We worked it out. We had never been super invested in monogamy, so it was not as big of a deal for us as it might have been for some other people.

The first thing I did was to talk to John about it. I called him up, because I had his number you see (laughing), and asked him to meet me in [a neighboring part of town].

John: I was stunned, I thought he wanted to meet so he could knock my block off. Instead, we sit there having coffee and talking about Sara. It was really weird at first, but I slowly came to realize over the next few, the next couple of times we saw, I met him, that he really was OK with it and wanted the best for Sara.

We discussed the evolution of their triad for some time, with the three explaining how they evolved to a more comfortable state together. Eventually I asked, "So why is monogamy not a big deal for you?" and they responded:

Sara: Even from the beginning, we had trysts with other people. I remember at our wedding I was taking the best man, Cal's good friend, up to the roof to have sex with him and when we got there, Cal and one of the bridesmaids were already there. He was like, oops, pulling up his pants. We all laughed about it and went back downstairs.

Cal: It is also where we live. The Bay Area is really free, sexually open compared to most places, so it was easier and lots of people just kind of went with it. Our friends didn't think it was a big deal either, well, some of our friends. Others were more monogamous, but even so . . .

John: It actually had been a big deal for me, and my ex-wife. Neither of us were "faithful" [air quotes] and we both used it against the other, so we weren't really monogamous but we fought about it a lot.

> Elisabeth: So Sara, if monogamy is not a big deal, why not just tell
> Cal that you wanted to have an open relationship? Why not just be
> direct from the get go?
>
> Sara: I have wondered that myself, and I have to say I don't really
> have a good answer for that. It just kind of happened, I didn't plan it,
> I didn't even really know it was fully happening until it kind of al-
> ready started, I just kind of found myself doing it. Really, I wish I had
> a better answer for you, but there it is.

This relationship, begun by happenstance and not negotiated, was one of the few that I observed continuing beyond the initial attempts to slide from monogamy to polyamory.

In addition to having a flexible attitude toward monogamy—something that is crucial for polyamorous relating—one of the main reasons that the Bayside triad was able to make the transition from affair to triad was because of the emotional health of Sara and Cal's relationship. Sara's deception regarding her relationship with John was an isolated incident, Cal had loved and felt loved by Sara for many years, and he was confident enough in himself not to be completely undone by his wife's desire for another man. If this was simply another in a long string of lies and cheating from Sara, or had Cal been more jealous or emotionally excitable, things would have most likely turned out quite differently. As it was, Sara told the truth the vast majority of the time, and as a result Cal trusted her, and Cal was an extraordinarily calm and thoughtful person. In fact, John sees Cal's equanimity as advantageous to his relationship with Sara, even beyond its calming effect when Cal did not "knock his block off." John reported that

> Sara and I are both kind of high strung sometimes, a little more
> reactive, a little bit wooooaaaaa occasionally. Cal though, he is solid.
> He can calm us both down and help us communicate. I can think of
> at least two different times we would have broken up if Cal hadn't
> been there to help us talk it out. He keeps us grounded, helps us
> work it out. He really is an amazing guy.

Cal's calm personality, both men's ability to accept open relationships, and John's reciprocal willingness to connect emotionally with Cal enabled the three to become friends, rather than rivals or enemies. The men clearly admired each other and loved Sara deeply.

For her part, Sara reported being

> completely blissed out. Things are good and have pretty much always been good with Cal, we are really good together, and that is super stable. John, on the other hand, is a little flighty, more intense, and as kinky as a cheap garden hose. So I get to explore new areas of myself with him, try new things that maybe Cal is not that into, and just be a different person with him . . . And the sex is great. It takes both of 'em to keep up with me [laughing]. Just the other week we were out for afternoon coffee. The girls [Sara and Cal's sixteen-year-old daughter, and John's eighteen-year-old daughter] were out some-where, doing their thing, and we had "slept late" [air quotes] and walked down the block to get some coffee. We were cuddled up in the booth together, both men kind of petting me or touching me, and the guy at the table across the way said "You look like you're happy" and I had to smile because I really was. So we must have just been radiating our satisfaction, for this guy to notice it, but yeah, things are great, they are really really good. I am grateful every day for the wonderful men in my life.

Cal, John, and Sara found that a relationship begun in dishonesty can still thrive if other elements of it—honesty in most areas, trust, love, a mutual commitment to work it out—are stable and functioning posi-tively.

The Veto Trap

Eventually Rick responded to two online ads—the first time either of us initiated a search for an additional partner rather than simply discussing it. Rick's Internet dating was unsuccessful, and his pursuit of it was lukewarm at best. During this phase, I requested that we institute a "veto policy" in which either one of us could ask the other to stop seeing someone if we felt that the other person was a threat to our family. At that point we both thought the veto was to help me feel more comfort-able with any girlfriends with whom Rick might become emotionally intimate.

Characteristic of newbie mistakes and couple privilege, many poly relationships have foundered on the impact of the veto. In our case, I was the one who pushed to include veto power in our agreement because I wanted Rick to keep his ultimate loyalty with me and the kids. In other cases, men are the ones who stipulate or use the veto, and for still other relationships both partners occasionally implement veto power. Among most long-term polyamorists, however, the existence and use of the veto is a red flag signaling couple privilege, insecurity, and poor relationship skills. In our case, the veto was initially a symptom of my insecurity with polyamory and my place in the relationship with Rick. At root, the assumption that the couple relationship should supersede all others and be protected at all costs is definitional to couple privilege, and so the veto becomes emblematic of the couple's ultimate ability to preserve itself.

Rigid rules in general can in fact be a sign of couple privilege in that they usually function to preserve the sanctity of the couple relationship. Tacit Campo commented that

> I talk to people all the time about relationship structures, and every time it comes down to things like veto power or rules-based relationships I always hear the same defense: "Well, if all the people involved are happy, what's wrong with it?" Thing is, I don't know that I've *ever* seen anyone with this approach to relationship who is actually happy. "Not feeling jealous right at this moment in time as long as the rules are followed" isn't the same thing as "happy."

Rather than a veto power and other rules, practiced polyamorists tend to rely on each others' good judgment, ability to work through difficulties, and positive regard for each other. Phoenix and Zack found that, after many years together:

> Zack: We didn't need a lot of rules with each other. We know each other well enough and trust each other to have our best interest at heart, so rules are pretty much moot at this point. We simply lead our lives in accordance with what works best for us and our relationship, and that tends to be a fairly consistent thing. If something comes up we talk about it, but usually there is rather little we need to negotiate now. We've been doing this long enough that we know what we're doing.

> Phoenix: A lot of it is just common sense. We don't have to have a lot of rules about who sleeps where and what kinds of sex we can have because we are aware of each other's needs and boundaries. And we

know we practice safer sex anyway, so we don't have to rehash it all the time.

While he disavowed rules in general, Tacit later acknowledged that there were some rule-ish kinds of things that could structure poly relationships.

Common rules that I have seen in real-world healthy poly relationships among happy people . . . tend to be few . . . The ones I tend to see include:

- Communicate openly.
- Be honest.
- Negotiate safer-sex arrangements and make sure everyone is in the loop about changes to sexual status.
- Be compassionate.
- Take responsibility for yourself and your actions, including the unintended consequences of your actions.
- Be flexible.
- Don't be a dick.

Rather than an externalized list of detailed rules, these experienced polys used an internally directed approach, applying their ethical perspectives to the situation of the moment. Above all, "Don't be a dick/Be compassionate" to your partners and other people is the primary ethic underlying these poly structures, and the others flow from there. As Cliff put it, "It's not about controlling the behaviors of other people with rules, it's about how not be a dumbass."

COMPLETE MEMBERSHIP

Gradually I took on a complete group membership role, meaning that I had a polyamorous relationship and thus became a community "insider." It is only in retrospect that I see this transition; at the time everything was so murky that I did not identify a specific moment or incident in which Rick and I became polyamorous or I adopted a poly identity.

Friendship with Steve

My friendship with Steve began during this time, over a year after I had
interviewed him. At that time we had acknowledged mutual intellectual
interests during the interview and discussed seeing each other socially,
but neither pursued it. Steve heard that I had returned home through
the polyamorous grapevine, emailed me, and we discussed spending
time together socially. He lived nearby and came over one evening for a
spur-of-the-moment walk with me, Rick, and the kids. We quickly began seeing each other several times a week. I was fascinated by his
sharp mind and charmed by his wit, and I was well accustomed to
becoming friends with people related to my research and thought that
my relationship with Steve would fall into the well-worn groove created
by my numerous platonic relationships with local polyamorists.

Steve began to drop by to help me in the morning, a time of day that
had proved particularly onerous for me as I tried to get myself ready for
work and the kids fed and dressed. Even more important than his
assistance, Steve's companionship was wonderful for me. Recent difficulties with other friends had left me in search of additional friendship
and support, and my friendship with Steve met those needs, rapidly
becoming increasingly emotionally intimate. Initially, Rick and Steve
enjoyed spending time together. Rick and I would have Steve over for
dinner, walks, park outings, movies, and late-night conversations. Our
time together as a group usually included our infant and toddler, who
quickly came to see Steve as another one of his adult friends (the infant
was too young to articulate the concept of a friend). Within several
weeks, however, Rick and Steve began to irritate each other. Steve
arrived for his morning visits after Rick had already departed for work,
so Steve and I spent far more time together independently than the
three of us did as a group. Rick became increasingly alarmed at the
growing bond between Steve and me.

Roughly two weeks after we began seeing each other as friends,
Steve said that he had fallen in love with me. "I didn't mean to," he
reported. "It just happened." I was shocked. I was just getting to know
him and already he was in love with me? I wondered if it were true, and
why he moved so quickly. I told him I liked him a lot and would like to
continue to spend time with him, but I did not, even now, think of
myself as a polyamorous person and was really seeking a platonic

friendship. Steve was confused by my lack of polyamorous identification and pointed out that Rick and I were in an open relationship. I replied that yes, Rick and I were in an open relationship, but I had never intended to become romantically involved with others. Steve's confusion remained, but he agreed to a continued friendship. Rick was displeased by Steve's admission and relieved that I did not return Steve's feelings.

Rick's Polyamorous Relationship

At this same time, Rick had a short fling with Joya, a good friend of ours from the local polyamorous community. We had socialized regularly with her and her son, and our children had become friends. Joya also provided paid childcare for us for several months, watching our children so I could write. She and I routinely attended numerous women's support group meetings together. Joya was also homeless (or as she preferred, a "postmodern Gypsy") for much of this time, staying with various lovers, friends, or her ex-husband. She would sleep on our couch once a month or so, sometimes more. She had a key to our house, and she knew she was free to come in whenever she wished.

Very late one night, Joya dropped by on her way home from work to pick up something she had left at our house. The house was dark, and she thought everyone was asleep. She let herself in to silently retrieve her belongings and depart. Instead, she found Rick and I snuggled on the floor in a pile of pillows with a bottle of wine. Joya joined us on the cushions where we snuggled and chatted. I became uncomfortable as the snuggling took on a decidedly more erotic tone. My stomach began to ache, and I realized that I was just not comfortable having a threesome that night, if at all.

I excused myself, saying I was exhausted because it was three a.m. and I had been up since six a.m. the previous day. Rick came into our bedroom to see if I was okay. I replied that I was fine, I was tired, and I did not want to have sex with Joya. He should, I informed him, go back into the living room and have sex with her. She was clearly open to it, and I wanted Rick to finally try polyamory so we could finally settle the issue.

Rick was hesitant, but after some discussion, he returned to Joya in the living room. I briefly anticipated lying awake, nervously listening or feeling uncomfortable. Then I immediately went to sleep and did not awaken until I felt Rick and Joya join me later. I moved over and the three of us slept for the rest of the night.

I awoke last the next day, amazed to find myself nonchalant about the whole incident. Joya, off to work hours before, had left a note asking me to call her and tell her how I was feeling. Rick called from work to check in, and I informed him of what I found to be a surprising lack of reaction. I kept waiting for the onset of insecurities and jealousy I had feared for these many years, and they never came. I surprised myself by feeling just fine about it, and I began to think that I might be able to do this, after all. Granted, Joya had been a close friend for several years and I trusted her. I knew that she respected me and would never try to get Rick to leave me for her. After that night, Rick and I continued to socialize with Joya. Rick and Joya only had one more sexual encounter while I was out of town. After that, neither Rick nor Joya put much effort into arranging additional sexual liaisons, and both expressed to me that they were less interested in each other as individual lovers than as components of a trio that included me.

Joya already knew Steve through connections in the local polyamorous community, and she began to socialize with him at the house Rick and I shared with our children. Joya, Steve, Rick, and I spent a few late nights together, sitting around the kitchen table discussing polyamorous life and our relationships. During one of these late-night kitchen conversations I expressed some dissatisfaction with a long-term communication pattern in which Rick and I routinely engaged. Steve and Joya held views similar to mine, and Rick began to feel "ganged up on" when they both intoned their opinions. After a series of negative communication, the relationship between Rick and Joya deteriorated to almost nothing.

Initially, the relationship between Joya and Steve was cautious. As they came to know each other, they established a friendship and ultimately united in their common opposition to Rick. Concurrently, Rick had a series of negative experiences that changed his mind regarding the desirability of polyamorous relationships. Joya's anger and rejection mystified and alarmed him. In California, Jonathan discovered Theresa's ongoing adultery and filed for divorce. Rick worried that the introduction of the idea of multiple partners into their relationship had spurred Theresa's infidelity, and that the two might still be married were it not for our discussions of polyamory. Most importantly, Rick did not like Steve and was becoming increasingly uncomfortable with my friendship with him. The combination of these factors spurred Rick's rising unease with the practice of polyamory.

I Fell in Love with Steve

Soon after the night of the argument in the kitchen, Rick asked me to make an appointment with him so we could discuss our relationship during the day, with no children present. I agreed and we arranged for my mother to spend time with the children that coming Saturday so Rick and I could talk. Coincidentally, Rick, Steve, and I had arranged a few weeks before to go dancing with several other polyamorous friends that Friday night, the night before the scheduled discussion. Rick asked that we refrain from serious conversation regarding our relationships that night and just "have fun," and I agreed.

That Friday evening during the dancing I felt a significant shift and realized I was in love with Steve. Steve could tell something had just happened and wanted to know what it was and so, even though Rick had requested a night free of serious conversation, the three of us left the dance club and took a walk. Rick requested some time alone with me before I told them both what was on my mind and, characteristic of couple privilege that relegates secondary partners to a secondary class in service of maintaining the couple relationship, we asked Steve to give us a moment. Steve went away for fifteen minutes, and Rick reminded me of our conversation date for the next day. He confessed that he had been planning to ask me to abandon polyamory in favor of a monogamous relationship. Initially I was stunned, aghast that both events (his desire to quit polyamory and mine to engage in it) should happen at once. Then I became irate, livid at what I perceived to be Rick's constant harassment of me to engage in polyamory for ten years and then his rapid reversal as soon as it was a man with whom I wanted to have a relationship rather than the woman Rick had envisioned all these years. Steve returned and I told him I loved him, but that Rick did not want us to be together. Steve was very angry with Rick and yelled at him briefly before I stepped between them. In our continued discussions over the next several days Rick explained that he was not necessarily requesting that I forgo polyamory completely, only a relationship with Steve specifically, whom he found increasingly problematic. I replied that Steve was the only person I had been even remotely interested in over the many years of interaction with numerous potential suitors, and that I was not interested in polyamory in the broad sense but in a relationship specifically with Steve.

Rick effectively "vetoed" Steve, asserting his desire that Steve and I discontinue any form of relationship. While I had initially been the one to request a veto policy in order to protect my relationship with Rick, when the time came that it was my relationship that was being vetoed I balked, arguing that he had bullied me into polyamory in the first place. Those agreements I had made with him were not valid, I argued, because they were made under duress and thus not binding. Rick felt betrayed by my refusal to honor such a foundational element of our agreement, especially when he had agreed to it at my behest. I felt betrayed by what seemed to me his willingness to sacrifice years of my emotional comfort in order to have access to outside partners, only to suddenly reverse his position once it appeared that it was I, and not he, who might have multiple lovers.

180-Degree Turn About

Rick and I had switched places: now I wanted to have a poly relationship with both him and Steve, and Rick wanted to be monogamous. Common to other newbie disasters, the way the relationship ended up working out was far different than either of us had imagined, and we had a hard time adapting to it. With what in retrospect appears to be eerie prescience, Joya Starr told me in her initial interview in 1997:

> It is a poly phenomenon that often the woman in the couple is kind of reluctant and is dragged kicking and screaming into poly. Then when the man is done with his experimentation, the woman often finds that it suits her character and stays with it. It is almost like acquiring a skill, once she's got it, it becomes part of how she wants to live her life. It can be real confronting when the man wants to become involved in the poly lifestyle and then finds out that it is really much easier for a woman to establish relationships, and not only do they establish them easier, they tend to get more intimate and deeper faster, cause that is what women are good at. Speaking

generally, women like that kind of stuff. So the men can become very uncomfortable.

Little did I know how accurate her prediction would be at the time and how closely my relationships with Steve and Rick would mirror the cliché "poly phenomena."

Things Fall Apart

Rick and I sought couple's counseling and found it effective in improving our communication, and I sought personal counseling. I tried to maintain a platonic friendship with Steve in order to give the men a chance to work out an amicable relationship, but when it became clear that they were never going to be able to share me in a friendly fashion, I "broke up" with Steve. At the end of that discussion, I kissed him goodbye, which turned out to be a big mistake. Previously untested sexual tension bubbled to the surface and we "made out" with the fervor of those who thought they would never see each other again.

By establishing an amorous relationship with someone from my research setting, I made the transition to a complete membership role characterized by full immersion in the scene as a "native" who shared a "common set of experiences, feelings, and goals" with those in my setting.[7] Ironically, it was at this transition to complete membership status that I disengaged almost completely from the local polyamorous community. I was overwhelmed with emotional discord and spent so much time in personal and couple's counseling and intense personal discussion with both men that I had no time left for community interaction.

Steve and I stayed broken up for two months, during which time I tried to forget about him and polyamory. I could not put him out of my mind, though, and six weeks into the breakup I initiated discussions with Rick regarding my desire to reunite with Steve. Rick and I had not yet reached agreement when I ran into Steve in public and began seeing him again. That time it lasted for a month. I could not tolerate the tension of being pulled between the men, so I again broke up with Steve.

During this tumultuous and painful period, my greatest concern was for my children. Rick and I tried to shield them from the fighting by having the discussions only late at night when they were asleep, a strategy that was proving increasingly difficult to maintain. We were exhausted by our late-night discussions, and our discord occasionally spilled over into daylight hours. Although the children were young enough to remain oblivious to the majority of the content of the arguments, they were still uncomfortable because they could feel the tension and could tell the adults were upset.

In the midst of this turmoil, I saw an adjunct job listing at university in a town where my sister and brother-in-law resided. I accepted the adjunct job, Rick and I sold our house, and we moved away from the area we had recently shared with Steve. While I wanted to be near my sister and the job offered the potential for a professional future, these incentives would not normally have been sufficient to spur me to quit my job, sell my house, and move my family to another state. The added impetus of my overwhelming desire to see Steve and the negative impact that had on my relationship with Rick drove me to drastic action.

Relationship Drama

The dramatic, almost soap-operatic tone my relationships took on at that point is characteristic of the worst of polyamory. Other respondents and their children routinely mentioned the drawbacks of emotional pain, complexity, and dramatic relationships as negative aspects of polyamory. Especially potent at first before newbies have had a change to practice managing jealousy or negotiating safer-sex agreements, the complexities inherent in this challenging relational style magnify relationship strengths and weaknesses, creating higher highs and lower lows for those involved.

This is not to say that all poly relationships are drama laden—much like monogamous relationships, there is tremendous variety in how people handle their multiple-partner interactions. In our case specifically, our high expectations and inability to shift our agreements with changing life and relationship circumstances made it very difficult to work things out smoothly. In other relationships, there is a marked lack of drama. Some people, especially those who have practiced for many years and established long-term poly relationships, have honed communication skills and crafted agreements that are low drama and low maintenance. They simply function, with normal family issues and no particular upheavals.

Both the Campo and Wyss families are exemplary of calm, nondramatic poly families. In each case, family members have gone through significant transitions with each other and the form of the family has shifted over time. Things happen in their family lives—the death of a spouse in a traffic accident, a traumatic brain injury, cross-country moves, divorce—and they use their skills to deal with it. They are not constantly freaked out; their family lives flow smoothly without recurrent drama. Tacit Campo explained the easy functioning of his family:

> You keep asking me how I deal with the complexity but I am really not finding my relationships all that complex. It is what it is, and it works well for all of us. The primary worry in our lives is financial because the farm is in such dire straits, that is where the tension comes from. And we deal with it as best we can, but things are good in many other ways. There is a marked absence of the drama and complexity I hear about in other poly relationships, I think because of how we handle ourselves and the fact that no one had to be talked into becoming poly.

A few adept polyamorists were able to manage these myriad pitfalls, but such navigation took skill reliably developed only through practice. The majority of polyamorists had at least some relationships filled with pain and drama, and they did not tend to continue with those relationships. Most often, they took what they learned about relationships, themselves, and their partners and went on to form other relationships with new people or deepen existing relationships. I do not discuss drama in depth here because drama is such a constant theme throughout the book that I am certain readers will have many opportunities to understand it in context.

WITHDRAWAL FROM THE POLY COMMUNITY

My disastrous relationship, moving to a new place, and the fact that I had completed the first wave of data collection all combined to propel me out of contact with the poly community. After our initial slow-motion disaster with polyamory, both Rick and I were wary of polyamory and focused instead on trying to strengthen our relationship with each other. For several years I did not collect any data on polyamory,

though I continued speaking on the research findings at academic conferences. Audience members would routinely ask the same questions—
"What about the children? How does this relationship style affect the
children?" While I could provide data from my years of participant
observation and watching poly families interact, I could not answer
questions about the children's thoughts, feelings, or experiences because I was not allowed to ask them questions. Over time I began to
wonder how my former respondents were doing and decided to see if I
could find out, embarking on the Longitudinal Polyamorous Family
Study.

Picking Up the Pieces

For the next five years Rick and I tried doggedly to heal the rift in our
relationship, attending couples counseling and both working hard to
nurture positive feelings for each other. While I missed Steve keenly, I
refrained from contacting him at that point and instead invested myself
in my work at a university and my family. I sought to deal with my
lingering angst with personal counseling, meditation, exercise, antide-
pressants, aromatherapy, chocolate, and pretending to be content.
Things did slowly improve, and over a period of about three years Rick
and I fought less and felt better about each other. I kept looking for
ways to fall in love with Rick again, change my desire to leave the
relationship, or at least manage to endure it more comfortably. Try as I
might nothing seemed to work, and I became increasingly despondent.
Three years into that cycle it became clear to me that our progress
toward a more intimate and positive relationship had ground to a halt,
and we stagnated in that steady state for two more years.

Splitting Up with Rick

By the time the children were five and seven, I could no longer tolerate
my distressingly leaden relationship and informed Rick that I wanted to
split up. We had both tried as hard as we could and, while our relationship was tolerable for him, I was miserable, and it did not appear to be
getting any better. Several months later I moved out, and we began to
share custody of the children, who stayed with him most of the time but
came to me regularly. Although the fact that we had tried so hard, told

each other the truth, and refrained from cheating on each other made it easier to continue to trust each other and collaborate as coparents, it was still a painful time. I tried to reestablish contact with Steve at that point, but he wanted nothing to do with me and I don't blame him, after the way Rick and I used couple privilege to try to protect our relationship at Steve's direct emotional expense.

Coparenting, Amicable Divorce, and Relationship Continuity

Characteristic of some polys whose romantic relationships implode but whose friendships are able to weather the transition, Rick and I focused on maintaining positive relations with each other so we could coparent with the least conflict possible. At times we have been good friends again, supporting each other and coming to each other's assistance in times of need. Other times we have fought because our issues did not magically resolve with the end of our romantic relationship. It is easier now, and ultimately we both want what is best for the other. This positive regard allows us to mingle comfortably at family events or school functions, and we both continue to interact with each other's extended families.

Melody Lupine reported a similar experience with maintaining positive relationships with both of her ex-husbands from her triad:

> We stayed really good friends and one of the things that polyamory really benefitted from was we didn't need to hire attorneys, we didn't do the battle, the custody thing, it was all agreed upon and we, I actually wrote up the divorce papers. We wanted what was best for the kids . . . and so I actually saw a real benefit from polyamory in the sense that I still loved this person and that's why we had gotten together in the triad. It wasn't about, just because something doesn't work out or things don't go right that you just hate this person and then, I think polyamory really gave me a view of, just because some things don't work out doesn't mean we have to become enemies and so we kept a good friendship through it. Definitely a positive related to polyamory, a benefit.

In fact, Melody was able to maintain such a positive relationship with Quentin that he routinely attended family functions such as birthdays and holiday dinners:

Quentin and I had a tumultuous time when we fought for custody of Zane and I moved out here. It got pretty ugly. We are in a loving relationship right now; he is very supportive. He even brought this up just this week with my birthday, saying how remorseful he was that things didn't work out with us. Anyway, life is interesting, that we can even express that to each other. So I know that even though there may be things you go through, you can still have this connection and keep it. Even though Quentin and I aren't in this romantic or sexual or intimate relationship, we still love each other, that love is still there . . . When we had a birthday party for Zane, we all went out to a family dinner. Quentin's part of the family, we go to all of Zane's soccer games together. My new partner went to his birthday party, and he's like "oh, you and Quentin sit together" and then we took pictures together and he's like "Wow, he's your ex!" When Pete graduated, Quentin went to the graduation. He's going to be at Joyce's graduation. He's family, very much so.

Melody related her ongoing connection with Quentin to their mutual willingness to work things out, something that was currently lacking in her relationship with Cristof, even though their initial divorce had gone well. I asked her how things had changed with her and Cristof, and she stated the following:

Elisabeth: So your relationship with Cristof, it sounds like, at some point, it went from you two having a relationship to your relationship being around his contact with the kids. Am I reading that correctly?

Melody: Yeah, when he got into a monogamous relationship, that is when things shifted in a lot of ways. With us, with the kids. You know, he came into this monogamous relationship that no longer included me, which was fine; I was fine with that. "Let's just still have a connection." But then it became about the kids, and when I would confront him about "Hey, your kids over here" then it got tenuous between us. As he got further and further away from his kids, now it's like, we don't talk at all.

Elisabeth: You just have no relationship at all with him now.

Melody: No. Because as the kids turned eighteen, both of them, I told him, when both of them turn eighteen, the relationship between you and your dad is between you two. When you were under eighteen I was the mediator in between, but now whatever you guys want to make it, that's up to you.

Elisabeth: So you've just stepped out?

Melody: Yeah.

Elisabeth: But you maintained a relationship with Quentin.

Melody: He was different. He moved out here. He kept saying, "I don't care how rough it is, I still want to stay connected to you and Zane." I think we had to go through that ugly custody battle thing to really get through some of our stuff. After that, he moved out here and kind of looked at what his priorities were. We keep a lot of personal distance, but it still works, absolutely.

Cristof's decision to pour all of his time and resources into his "new" family contrasted sharply with Quentin's decision to move to be closer to his child and coparent.

Now What?

For two years I barely dated, focusing on my work, children, and playing roller derby. I was very clear about my relationship priorities: My children were (and remain) my "primaries," meaning that I consider them first when I make decisions, allocate resources such as time or money, or face any significant life issues. Emotionally, my secondary relationship was with roller derby, and dating came in a distant third. Characteristic of both the polyamorous tendency to tailor relationships outside of conventional roles and the propensity for some single parents to prioritize their relationships with their children over dating, I invested myself most deeply in work, playing a sport, and platonic relationships with family and friends.

When I eventually did begin to date, I found that poly people regularly contacted me online, and the dating website routinely suggested matches with people who ended up being polyamorous. Unsure of what I wanted or how I felt, I did not (and still do not) identify as poly, but I did not demand or offer sexual exclusivity. I eventually dated several poly people, and I had fun with them but did not identify it as a polyamorous relationship on my end because I was not emotionally invested, and I was certainly not in love. My dates may have seen me as polyamorous, and even possibly defined me as a tertiary or even secondary partner, but we never had a "define the relationship" talk. In complex and shifting relationships, it is quite possible that different people will define the same relationship in quite different ways.

After five years of single life, sometimes dating and sometimes not, I established a deep emotional connection with "Ann." Reminiscent of my attitude when I was in love with Rick, I felt no desire to see other people and transitioned some other relationships to platonic friendships. Ann had not asked me to do so, and I am not sure if she even knew—the impetus to be sexually exclusive came from my own experience of emotional intimacy with Ann and lack of desire for sexual contact with others. While Ann and I were both aware of polyamory and thought that we might consider the possibility at some future point, we agreed easily to monogamy and maintained that throughout our relationship. Eventually we broke up for reasons completely independent of this research.

For the last year and a half I have been in a "monogamish" relationship with Kira, a woman I adore. We are monogamous in practice, with the flexibility to allow things to spontaneously happen with other people—the "make out with someone in a bar" pass. Like my previous experiences, I am finding that being in love with someone significantly dampens not only my desire for, but also even my awareness of, other people. While in theory either of us could have another partner (or at least a fling) at any point, neither of us are particularly interested in seeking other relationships. In a life that sometimes feels too busy with children and work, I have a limited amount of time and attention for relationships and want to focus on nurturing the one I already have.

In light of this experience, I have concluded that I both believe in and can practice polyamory, but I am not polyamorous by orientation. Because my sex drive is insufficient to meet even Kira's needs at this point, I always have a lot to do, I enjoy time alone, and above all I am devoted to my beloved. I am in no rush to establish additional relationships—or even make out with anyone in a bar. I am, however, happy to have the freedom to do so if I wish, and I am glad that Kira and I have agreed to such flexibility. Because I seem to prefer monogamy when I am emotionally invested, I do not identify as polyamorous. If there is one thing I have learned in my study of poly folks, it is that people and life circumstances change over time, and frequently things end up turning out quite differently than anyone would have anticipated. If at some point in the future my relationship status changes, then my identification may change as well.

Melody Lupine made a similar transition to monogamy after having been in polyamorous relationships for many years, though hers was far more intentional, where mine was experimental and accidental. Melody reported that she

> realized that I had not yet experienced a conscious monogamous relationship. When I was married to my husband [Cristof] for seventeen years it was very much unconscious and was doing it more out of healing and repeating patterns from my family of origin and learning stuff, and so now what I wanted to create was what I considered a conscious monogamous relationship because I haven't experienced that yet. And so that wasn't very much in line with polyamory, so it was very hard having this background of polyamory then to make a shift back into monogamy.

While Melody had already begun to grow increasingly "disheartened with pursuing a polyamorous lifestyle in the sense that I was looking for one committed relationship," she shifted more to conscious monogamy when she was diagnosed with a serious illness. In a support group session for women with life-threatening illnesses, Melody had an epiphany that the significant role she played in the national polyamorous community was not working for her because

> polyamory was no longer congruent with where my life was going and so I realized that I no longer wanted to be the spokesperson for the polyamorous community because I wasn't finding it working in my own life and that I had to represent a population who wasn't always doing poly the way I believed poly. Many people that were just cheating around and having affairs and saying "well, I'm poly," so after being so prominent in national leadership for about four or five years I was just, I realized it was not something I wanted to do any more.

Instead, Melody said that she wished to create a relationship based on conscious monogamy:

I think there is a level of depth and connection that I wanted to experience. When I say a conscious monogamous that wasn't there in the, just because I'm a different person than I was then and again its just what I am choosing to experience at this time in my life. I just want to take this relationship with this one person, see how much I can learn and grow and go deep with this one person. I know when you try to include more than one, I have unlimited love, so I have experience. But time and energy are limited resources, so with that, the more relationships you bring in, the less time and energy you have for each of them. I'm not saying that polyamory is bad or wrong, its just that right now that's not what's working in my life and what I choose to do, but its nice to know that it is a choice, because before it wasn't. Now I can choose monogamy, I can choose polyamory, I can choose to be heterosexual, I'm at choice. My choices can change.

One of the choices Melody saw as remaining a possibility was the potential for a flexible vision of monogamy:

I still consider myself polyamorous in my *views*, I am very poly *oriented*. I'm open, I'm not jealous. I can be open to sharing my partner under the right circumstances. Actually, in this conscious monogamy we have an agreement: For our sexual learning, like, my partner right now has never been with two women and him. I told him, with agreements, I would totally go into that situation to give him that experience. If that would be growing and learning for him, then I am not jealous. I am not afraid to enter that as a one-time experience. I would embrace that with a sister, as long as it didn't take anything away from the relationship and added something to it.

After coming to realize what I call the *polyamorous possibility*, or that it is possible to maintain happy and healthy, openly conducted, non-monogamous relationships, Melody retained inflections of those options, as well as the poly ethics of self-growth and rejection of jealousy.

Melody is unique among my respondents for a number of reasons, and especially germane to this section are her prominence in the national polyamorous community in the United States and her willingness to participate in the follow-up study. Of the fifteen respondents I was able to find from my first wave of data collection, Melody was the only person who had become monogamous and still chose to respond.

JEALOUSY AND COMPERSION

Jealousy is a significant issue in polyamorous relationships, and poly community members spend quite a bit of time and effort thinking and talking about jealousy. *Compersion* is a word polyamorists made up to describe the opposite of jealousy, or the feeling poly people get when they observe their partners happily in love with someone else. While some people anticipate being jealous, others are surprised by their own reactions.

Because polyamory can be so complex and surprising, many people anticipate their multiple-partner relationships working out differently in their imaginations than the actual relationships do in real life. In my case, this translated into my virtual certainty that I would be uncomfortable and jealous if Rick had other partners, and his virtual certainty that he would not experience jealousy of me and my imagined girlfriend. What actually happened surprised us both: I was not at all jealous of Rick's tryst with Joya, and Rick was quite jealous of my interactions with Steve.

James Majek discussed the common polyamorous event that a secondary partner is not jealous of the primary partner but becomes jealous if his or her partner establishes a relationship with another secondary. When Morgan began dating Nash, James reported that he

> had a meltdown . . . Well, I had just the classic jealousy reaction. No anger, just freaking out thinking or feeling like I was going to lose this person [Morgan]. I think it's the standard fear that if someone else gets into this other person's life, that they're going to find out that this other person is better and I'm going to lose.

Elisabeth: But you didn't feel that way with Clark?

James: When he started dating my wife [Melissa]? No, not really.

Elisabeth: Or even around Morgan? Because, what, he was already there?

James: See, that's what's interesting to me is that I never once had the slightest bit of jealousy around Clark because I see him as an integral part of the relationship that I have with Morgan because it's not just her, it's everything that comes with her. It's him; it's her kids. So to me, I want them [Morgan and Clark] to be doing well because when they're doing well, Morgan and I are doing well . . . with Clark and Melissa, as opposed to Morgan and Nash, I had just been with Melissa for so much longer. We've been married about ten, but together about eighteen years now. To me, there was a very mature relationship already in place. I didn't feel like this was a huge threat because we were talking about it seriously and openly . . . It's a kind of relationship that I consider rock solid and stable, difficult at times, but we really know each other. My relationship with Morgan is younger, more uncertain. If all of this happened within two years of Melissa and I being together, I think I would have freaked out because it's too uncertain. Here all of a sudden someone else comes along, what the fuck is this going on now? With Morgan it was "OK, I'm not settled in what we have yet. I don't know where this is going." So to have someone else coming in scared the shit out of me in a way it didn't with Melissa.

Characteristic of polyamorous community experience and rhetoric, James identified differing types of and reasons for jealousy, connecting it with uncertainty and fear of loss. What provoked jealousy with Morgan was unproblematic with Melissa because James felt more secure in the durability of his marriage and the clarity of his communication with Melissa than he did in his relationship with Morgan. In this and many other instances, jealousy proves situational and dependent on the specific tenor and interactions of the people involved.

Polyamorists also identify specific scenarios that can provoke jealousy and detail strategies to manage those situations. One recurrently problematic scenario involves one partner in an open couple with children establishing a relationship with a new person. Common poly community wisdom identifies New Relationship Energy or NRE as a booby trap of jealousy. NRE is the exiting, almost effervescent feeling one gets at the beginning of a positive relationship in which everything the other person says is new and fascinating, before reality and mundanity tarnish the exciting glow of perfect possibility. Unless they anticipate and compensate for the phenomena, people in the thrall of NRE are likely to neglect their longer-term partners in favor of the excitement of a new relationship. Colette—a white project manager in her late thirties—

described how she might react if her husband, Bruce, became enamored with someone else:

> Yeah, I could totally see being jealous if he hooked up with someone he really dug and they ended up having lots of dates and I took care of the kids all the time. I love him and I want him to be happy, and I really do want to be poly, but I just don't want to be stuck at home eating mac and cheese with the kids while he is out eating steak with his new flame. Right now we are both kind of dating a little bit but neither of us is serious with anyone else. For the dating, though, we make sure things even out, so if I am home with the kids in a week when he has a date after work then he makes sure to take them somewhere on the weekend so I can take a break or have lunch with a friend or whatever, date or not, just I have some time for myself, and vice versa. It is not tit for tat, not like I get a date and he gets a date, but more like we are both aware of how much personal time and time with the kids we each get. So if I ever did end up eating mac and cheese with the kids while he is at [local restaurant] with a hottie then it would be OK because I can have my own hottie, or a weekend in Vegas with the girls, or whatever, just, he recognizes that my time is important too. I know things are even in the long run so I don't really keep track.

In that same interview, Colette mentioned her confidence in the durability of her relationship and the couple's love for each other as a "secure bond" as additional reasons that she did not tend to feel jealousy. She and Bruce negotiated accommodations so that the event that Colette imagined would provoke jealousy—being "stuck at home eating mac and cheese with the kids while he is out eating steak with his new flame"—was defused by the explicitly acknowledged equity that deemed both partners equally worthy of personal time for dating or other things.

Discussing his strategy for dealing with NRE in his long-term relationship with Summer, Zack Phoenix (the person who actually coined the term *NRE*) said:

> I think of it as compensating for the wind in archery. If you are aiming for a target 50 yards away and the wind is blowing from the left, you angle your bow in to the wind a little bit so the arrow flies in an arc and still hits the target, even though the wind has been push-

ing on it. The same thing with a long-term partner, if you have this exciting new person you have just started seeing and you are really excited about them, then make sure to make a date night with your person over here, the one who might not be as exciting in the moment, not quite as new and shiny, but you love her and you have deep ties with her that need to be nurtured too. So bring her flowers, take her out to dinner, go away for the weekend together. Just don't get so blinded by the new that you forget to take care of the long-term relationships in your life.

In addition to overcompensating for the potential to ignore a long-term partner, polys also council each other to make plans or seek emotional support when a partner is out on a date. Billy Holestrom experienced the discomfort of remaining at home alone while his wife, Megan, and her boyfriend Jack went to a concert. Prior to their departure Billy had assured Megan and Jack that he was fine at home, he had a lot to do, and they should go have fun. Megan and Jack hesitated, offered to find a babysitter and to give Billy the spare ticket they had purchased prior to finding out that Billy did not want to attend the concert. After receiving Billy's reassurances that he was fine staying at home with Megan and Billy's daughter, Ariel, Jack and Megan left for the show and were gone for hours. Meanwhile, Billy put Ariel to bed and

> proceeded to have a minor meltdown, moping around the house feeling so sorry for myself while they were out having fun. Wah wah (melodramatic crying sound). It wasn't that I didn't want them to have fun, it was just that I was lonely and bored and did not want to deal with the mountains of laundry that I had on my agenda for that evening. And the fact that they had invited me and made it clear that I could come with them only made it worse, I couldn't even blame them for my being upset at them going out without me. So from then on I either go with them or plan to have something of my own to do that is more fun than laundry while they're out having a good time. It works better that way, I get a lot less upset and they don't worry about me brooding at home while they're trying to have fun.

Poly folks also report using introspection, counseling, and conversations with supportive friends as tools to investigate the underpinnings of jealousy. People who express problems with jealousy on poly websites or in support groups are routinely instructed to seek the issue beneath the jealousy that is provoking such an uncomfortable emotion. Those discussions routinely evolve to include significant focus on insecurity, determining one's needs, and asking for those needs to be met. Among long-term poly folks, the presence of jealousy signals the need for some accommodations or strategies to manage the specific situation, rather than a signal that the situation provoking the jealousy should stop immediately because it is making someone uncomfortable.

GENDER

While being extremely unusual in some regards, the polyamorous families I studied were surprisingly gender conforming in many ways. When there was a full-time parent it was most often a woman, and it tended to be women who were the family schedulers and managers. Women in these families did most of the cooking and cleaning and child care. Not that men were completely uninvolved in household and child care—certainly the poly fathers involved in this study were at least as involved with their children as mainstream monogamous men, some of them were excellent cooks, and a few of the families had full-time dads at home.

Some of this gender conformity was due to financial constraints: Men still make, on average, more money than women, and these families were no exception. It makes sense for the lower-earning parent to stay home with the children, even when there are multiple parents. Other poly families reported that desire to parent or practicality of childbearing and nursing were decisive in determining who stayed home with children. While Leah Tree changed her schedule in response to bearing the trio's son Will far more than her husbands Bjorn and Gene changed their schedules, she did it because she wanted to breastfeed Will:

> Leah: I spend more time parenting because I am nursing, and my more flexible job makes that easier. I can work from home, and we even have a nanny who comes to the house to take over with Will. I work fewer hours with basically no impact on my post-doc because there is no set job schedule I have to meet. I can coordinate the lab from home and write papers. This is a choice for me because there is not a financial cost or cost to my career to be home so I can nurse . . .

all that said I also get a tremendous amount of support from the men. Especially at the beginning the men did everything, and Gene especially has been able to take flex time and be home one day per week, as well as taking three months off when Will came. So even though I spend a bit more time with Will, but it is not a big inequality and often related to nursing.

Gene: Leah is also more likely to be around on the weekends with Will and Bjorn and I are more likely to go do something for a few hours, but we arrange our schedules so that when Will is awake we can spend time with him. I can often work at home, and I usually get up really early to have time to work before others are awake, and then I can play with Will when he wakes up so Leah can pump and I get to be with Will before I go to work.

Bjorn: We have all done a great job of supporting each other, getting as much access to Will as we can, and balancing our personal needs so everyone gets what they need. We all do everything we can, given the limitations of our jobs and commutes.

Leah: Other than the nursing thing, the parenting and family life in general is fairly gender equitable. We each cook one night a week, and the dads usually do bath time because I spend all day with Will. Each parent feeds Will and I pump so Bjorn and Gene can give him bottles. The men put Will to bed and I do the naps throughout the day.

Gene: Usually one of us gets up to get Will in the morning and get him ready for the day—whoever is sleeping alone has the monitor and gets up to deal with Will. The dads sleep through the monitor unless Will is really screaming, but Leah hears the monitor, every little sound.

Leah: Now the monitor is wherever I am not, except if Gene goes out on a date then I take the monitor.

The inequity of Leah hardly ever being on baby-monitor duty all night does not seem to bother "the dads" because, as Bjorn said, "We like to have the time with Will." Upon further inspection, this seemingly traditional gender division of labor is revealed as a carefully thought-out balancing act in which each of the adults contributes what appears to them to be an effort roughly equivalent to that of the other two, and each of the three is satisfied with how much time they get with the baby and alone for personal needs.

UNPREDICTABILITY

The prevalence of divorce and extramarital birth indicate that people in serially monogamous relationships have unpredictable relationship outcomes, such as committing to a relationship for life and then changing their minds once it becomes clear it is not working out. Considering how difficult it can be for two people to manage a dyadic relationship, it is no wonder that some—especially younger or less seasoned—polyamorous relationships can face a higher degree of unpredictability. My findings indicate that the larger the relationship and the more people involved, the more likely it is to have partners change over time. In addition to the complexity that accompanies multiple-partner relationships, the relative lack of cultural role models demonstrating consensually nonmonogamous relationships means that poly people must either construct their own patterns or find role models in polyamorous communities. Such self-direction can provide freedom and unpredictability.

In my own case, Rick had a very clear idea of what kind of poly relationship he wanted and how that should work out. I was less clear about what I wanted and did not harbor my own plan for how things would work out except that it would involve my continued relationship with Rick. In both cases, the relationship ended up being quite different from what either of us expected. Rick expected a woman with whom we could both partner, and I found a man. I expected to feel jealous and insecure, Rick expected that he would not feel jealous, and both of us were wrong.

While some people like Rick plan and envision their poly relationships in fantastic detail, in other cases poly relationships happen *to* people, simply evolving from their existing social lives in a way that no one had anticipated. Those who plan, seek, and avidly envision a poly relationship prior to engaging in one may build an image of what the relationship will be, which might be profoundly different than they had anticipated.

Complexity and Drama

Emotions and issues can be magnified in poly relationships, which are thus more likely to produce extremes—the highs of being crazy in love with not only one person but two or more people, at the same time, who also love each other and have had a healthy child together, can be overwhelming. The lows can be equally extreme—having multiple relationships break up at the same time or a fluid-transfer accident that involves transmitting a sexually transmitted infection or unplanned pregnancy.

All of this emotional intensity and constant communication can become wearing for some people. Kristine, a white poly woman, student, and world traveler, confessed to me that she was feeling quite exhausted by poly relationships for a time.

> I haven't seen many successful poly relationships. I've seen poly relationships where one partner tries to be poly, because they don't want to lose the other partner. I've seen women living in fear for years—afraid their husbands will leave them for someone younger, cuter, perkier . . . I've seen botox, and tears. I've heard people who had been in the poly community leave because they could no longer handle the stress and uncertainty, and I've heard people refer to poly as a graduate program in love. It can be a grueling fast lane to self-awareness, a long trip through hell, and moments of complete ecstasy. I don't advocate it. It isn't enlightened, it is complicated . . . and I've seen it bring joy, and pain.

Even though Kristine had previously been in a vee/sometimes triad with Evelyn and Mark Coach and was seeing two other people at the time of the interview (one of whom was engaged to be married to another woman), she was still not sure if she wanted to be polyamorous.

> I still wonder whether poly is worth the time, energy, and bandwidth, or whether it is just too rough on my self-esteem and emotions. The processing gets tiresome, and at the end of the day, wouldn't it be nice to simply be chosen, and cherished, and be the "most" whatever he loves me for being the "most" of? Who knows, maybe once I had my own primary, and felt safe, I would want to open things, maybe as a couple I'd be open to finding other couples. Two men one woman was lovely [grin]. But one thing is for sure—I

would have to think long, and hard, and have some serious talks about commitment [before having a child in a polyamorous relationship]. The CHILD would have to be our partnership's first priority, before I would do poly and children, because NO child will do well as an afterthought.

While Kristine reported that her poly relationships had spurred tremendous personal growth for her at various points, their high-maintenance communication and emotional styles came at such a high cost that she was not sure if the growth was worth it to her.

Experienced polyamorists know that polyamorous relationships with those new to polyamory, termed *newbies* or *first timers*, can potentially end catastrophically. Because of this risk, many long-time polys shy away from dating new polyamorists, who are more likely to revert to monogamy once the inevitable complexities of polyamorous relationships begin to take a toll.

Emmanuella Ruiz related her concerns regarding her new lover, whom she called "theoretically poly":

Poly in the abstract, no experience, no context. And in fact has a jealous streak a mile wide, something he didn't recognize until he met me and started having to face the reality of polyamory, so yeah. For him I think it is still very much in the abstract. I think he is a man of one heart. I do not think he is poly, I don't. Some people love one person. I think he's, I know he is polysexual. He's more than happy to be involved sexually with others, but he won't love more than one person, and the idea that I might love someone else threatens him.

While Emmanuella said she was definitely in love with him, she worried that their relationship might not make it because "I *am* poly; it is just what I am." She was concerned that they might not be able to maintain a long-term romantic relationship if he could not accept what she viewed as her "relational orientation." In that case, he might be a fly-through while she remained polyamorous.

Nori, a forty-nine-year-old small business owner with an adult child spoke of the regret she felt because she was in love with Lindsey, her girlfriend of a year and a half. Although Nori had been clear from their first meeting that she was polyamorous, Lindsey still wished them to be monogamous:

In the beginning of our relationship the poly thing was just a conversation and you'd talk about it and it seemed, like, OK, because it was in the distance and nothing very real was happening. And then the more we talked about Jorge the more she just didn't want to hear anything about him, didn't want to meet him, nothing. And it's just gotten worse. So now I'm having a great big bout of, oh my God, don't get involved with anybody who's not poly, who doesn't come from that orientation from the center!

Tacit Campo reiterated this point with tongue planted firmly in cheek when he said, "Poly newcomers tend to make the same mistakes, and I'd like to think that at this point in life, I'm ready to explore the exciting world of advanced, sophisticated relationship mistakes that waits beyond that field."

Even practiced polyamorists who fall in love with "monos" occasionally forget community wisdom and attempt to convert someone who was formerly monogamous to become polyamorous—sometimes successfully and sometimes with disastrous results. Poly people in smaller communities or more rural areas are more likely to attempt to convert a monogamous person to polyamory, though such attempts are less common in places with larger communities and many more potential partners who already identify as poly.

STIGMA

In this section I discuss my own experiences of poly-related stigma and relate them to the stigma respondents report encountering, using the concepts of *sex negativity* and the *polyamorous possibility* to explain the fear, suspicion, and hypersexualization that polys can experience in their social environments. I discuss respondents' experiences of stigma in relationship to families in far greater detail in chapter 7.

I experienced the stigma of polyamory, both personally and professionally. "Margaret," a close friend since childhood, stopped socializing with me because, she told me years later, she was "sick to death of always hearing about the poly thing. It seemed like it always came up in conversation, every single time I hung out with you and Rick." Other than Margaret, I have not been aware of any other friends rejecting me for attempting polyamory. My family has been similarly supportive, especially my mother and sister.

Professionally, the stigma of studying a sexual minority group—and worse (in some people's eyes) becoming one of "them" myself—was far more damaging than was the stigma in my personal life. Two separate Institutional Research Boards required gymnastic application processes with extremely time-consuming and absurd restrictions about the research records I was allowed to retain and the informed consent procedures I was required to follow.[8] While my open-minded dissertation chair was extremely helpful and provided excellent mentoring, other members of my dissertation committee were less able to compartmentalize their prejudice and acted unprofessionally during and after my dissertation defense.

Publishing has also been challenging. Journals related to sexualities have always been receptive to research on polyamory but are unfortunately ghettoized as second rate in the political world of academic sociology. Mentors like the chair of my department encouraged me to publish in "more diverse" (read mainstream) journals that spoke to the "core of the discipline" in order to gain tenure and be promoted to an associate professor. Unfortunately, editors and reviewers at many of the more mainstream journals had negative reactions to the topic itself, and I was routinely required to offer additional explanations and documentation that editors did not request from colleagues studying other topics.[9]

Finally, it was extremely challenging to identify grants appropriate to fund my research, something that became increasingly important as the worsening economic climate at the end of the 2000s forced universities across the United States to slash budgets and require faculty to find external resources to fund their own salaries, teaching assistants, and contribute financially to the university. Most grants were designed to support the study of mainstream families, and those dedicated to sexual minorities usually targeted gay and lesbian families. Additionally, grants targeted to "alternative" families often focused on abuse, molestation, drug use, and other negative family outcomes—issues I did not see appearing in my data. If respondents had reported these issues I certainly would have pursued them, but I was not about to manufacture them in order to get grants. Failing to secure external funding contributed significantly to my inability to gain tenure, and the narrowness of funded grant topics made it almost impossible for me to attain that funding. Sex negativity contributed to narrowing that field of potential topics and cast research related to sexual minorities as fringe enough to be irrelevant. As we shall see in chapter 10, this research has tremendous relevance for other families beyond those of polyamorists.

Sex Negativity, the Polyamorous Possibility, and Fear

This general attitude of fear, disdain, and suspicion, coupled with the relegation of sexuality to a sphere apart from legitimate social discourse, is what some scholars have termed *sex negativity*.[10] It was evident during my dissertation defense, dealings with IRBs, and editors' and reviewers' comments: sexuality is at once dismissed as a valid topic while simultaneously being held to different and higher standards than other topics. Were I to study monogamous, heterosexual families I would be viewed as a *family* researcher because I focus on family issues such as division of labor, parenting, interactions with institutions, and relationships with families of origin. In other words, my research does not focus on sexuality per se in that I am not asking my respondents about sexual positions or the mechanics of group sex. This study has focused on intimate partner and family relationships, much the same way other family studies have done. But the fact that my respondents are sexual/relational nonconformists brands the entire family style as hypersexual and me as a *sexuality* researcher. Such one-dimensional thinking that can see no farther than the sexual relationship is further evidence of sex negativity.

Among forms of sexual nonconformity, polyamory is unusual in that it could potentially be appealing to everyone who desires to have intimate relationships with other people. Most people are heterosexual, and it is readily apparent that not every one experiences same-sex sexual attraction or desire.[11] In other words, not everyone has the capacity or desire to be gay, lesbian, or bisexual. However, most people in marriages or other long-term relationships, regardless of sexual orientation, have had the experience of being attracted to someone else besides their partner. As such, almost everyone has the potential to be polyamorous in a way that they do not have the same potential to be gay. Once people become aware of the potential to negotiate openly conducted, nonmonogamous relationships, whether or not they actually wish to engage in them, they have realized the *polyamorous possibility*, and they can never unthink it again. They may reject the idea or decide to explore it further, but the potential for themselves or their partner to initiate discussion of a polyamorous relationship exists in a way it had not before they became aware of polyamory as a social option. Because the polyamorous possibility is potentially open to everyone, it is more threatening to mainstream society than are bisexual, gay, or lesbian relationships that require the (rarer) presence of same-sex desire.

It is this almost universal potential that links the polyamorous possibility so strongly to fear in some people's minds. This fear can be especially potent for those with unresolved infidelity issues in their own lives, as I experienced with my friends and committee members: Margaret told me about the deep pain she experienced when her mother and mother-in-law were both abandoned (respectively) by her father and father-in-law for younger women, and she expressed feelings of profound insecurity when she considered any scenario in which her husband might date someone else. One of the women on my dissertation committee had a nasty divorce several years earlier when she discovered her then-husband cheating on her with another woman. It is possible that journal editors or members of IRBs had similar personal issues that were enflamed by hearing about polyamory as well. Alternately, it is also possible that they were simply put off by the topic, or that they did not approve of my scholarship, writing, or conclusions. The specific tone of the reviews and recurrent nature of the negative feedback signals a deeper, institutionalized issue of sex negativity. Every writer gets critiques, but not every critique is so defensive and vitriolic in tone.

Respondents reported being held in suspicion when others in their social environments learn of their polyamorous relationships. Jana Founder reported that she was at a party for her son's graduation from kindergarten when another mom in attendance realized that Jana was polyamorous:

> It was ridiculous, she clung on to her husband with both hands and never took her eyes off me, as if I might just steal him out from under her nose. And my dance card is full, I have no room and no desire for any more partners. I am in no way a threat to her relationship, but clearly she saw me as a threat, much more so than my husband who is also polyamorous and was there with me. She never

really looked at him, but kept her eyes glued to me in a way that made me really uncomfortable. It was creepy, really. Obviously something was up for her, she must have some insecurity in her relationship or maybe she cheated on him or whatever, but it came across as somehow my fault or something. It was weird. We had never met before but she zoned right in on me once she knew, I was on her radar.

That feeling of suspicious surveillance was common among polys that came out or were outed in conventional, ostensibly monogamous social settings.

Buffers to Discrimination

One major difference between lesbigays and polyamorists is that the mainstream public is relatively oblivious to polyamory, with poly people remaining virtually invisible to society at large. Whether they embrace, despise, or are indifferent to lesbigays, almost everyone in the United States today is aware of the existence of lesbians, gay men, and (to a lesser extent) bisexuals. The same cannot be said of polyamorists, and this affords them a measure of protection from social stigma that is not as readily available to lesbigay people.

Because many in polyamorous relationships can legally marry in ostensibly monogamous, heterosexual dyads, they have different relationships with marriage than do most people in same-sex relationships. While lesbigays may also elect to marry someone of another sex in a similarly ostensibly monogamous and heterosexual dyad, it requires a far greater effort to maintain a closeted gay life than it would for polys with other-sex partners—a configuration that makes them socially intelligible as heterosexual couples with "close friends." This ability to remain closeted almost effortlessly is a resource to which many people in same-sex relationships do not have access and thus functions as a form of (often misattributed) heterosexual privilege that provides an easy buffer against effects of stigma against sexual nonconformists.

Is It Worth the Effort?

So was the challenge of my own poly relationship worth it to me? In retrospect, I think that if Rick and I had not tried polyamory we would not have split up. I certainly loved him enough to tolerate his wacky ideas, and he loved me. We were good companions with a lot in common who shared similar parenting styles and did not fight about money. Maybe it would have been best for us to eschew the whole mess. It certainly would have been better for Steve, who was extremely hurt by the entire episode. Alternately, Rick and I still might have split up even if we had never tried polyamory. Our miscommunication and power differences would have remained problematic for us regardless of our interactions with others. While it is possible that remaining monogamous (or even possibly poly in theory) would have placed less stress on our relationship issues, it is also possible that something else altogether would have happened. Polyamory did not create our problems, but our nonmonogamous relationships certainly exacerbated the problems we already had and created some new ones.

In addition to the pain and drama I experienced in what I came to think of as "the poly debacle" with Rick and Steve, I ended up learning a lot about myself and gaining some relationship skills that have been useful. I would not be the person I am today without those experiences. I am far more aware of my own motivations and behavior patterns, have much better boundaries, and am able to articulate my needs and emotions. Many poly people mention the potential for polyamory to spur self-knowledge and personal growth as a motivation for, element of, and outcome of polyamorous relationships. We will explore this idea in greater depth in chapter 8.

Impact on My Children

The children were so young during our family's brief and ill-fated poly episode that they were not aware of the implications of the adults' interactions at the time, and they had not established enough of a bond with Steve to miss his presence keenly the way they might have if they had been older. Rick and I were quite social, so our children were used to friends coming over and then going away: Steve's presence and absence blended in to the recurring parade of adults that passed through their social lives.

The tension that filled our lives, from a low background noise in daily family life to loud arguing, had a greater impact on the children than did Steve's presence or absence. Tension was a problem during "the poly debacle" and afterward as we tried to put our lives back together. Their parents' splitting up has been hard on my children, and they have felt many of the same fears and anxieties that most children feel when their parents separate. The overall positive tone that has characterized my coparental relationship with Rick helps to ameliorate some of their anxieties, and we have successfully modeled conflict resolution and ethical treatment. Less of the time, we have also modeled petty childishness and indignant outrage. The children have learned to consider boundaries, accept differences of opinion, flex with changing social circumstances, and gained a broader understanding of a wider variety of people as direct and indirect results of Rick and I experimenting with polyamory.

It has been challenging to know how exactly to discuss polyamory and our separation with our children. Several years ago I overheard the older child tell the younger child, "Mom and dad split up because mom had a boyfriend that dad didn't like." I was stunned and could not conceive of a way to tell them it was actually far more complicated than that, so I let the comment pass unremarked. They have accompanied me on research trips several times and overheard me discuss my research enough to know something of the broader story, and their understandings of it probably changed as they have matured. I am hoping they will eventually ask me what happened, but in the meantime I have not seen a good opportunity to discuss it that would not come across as bashing their dad.

I would have to say that, overall, polyamory has negatively affected my children and my life: My gut feeling is that it would have been better for all of us, and especially the children, if Rick and I had stayed together as a monogamous couple and never tried polyamory. Once we tried it and reacted as we did to a circumstance we had not anticipated, I was unable to trust Rick and move on, which made it impossible for me to remain in a romantic relationship with him. Polyamory can be high stakes—"playing with fire," as one respondent put it. For many it is well worth the risk, and for others like myself it is not. A different relationship with different people would have turned out quite differently, obviously, so I do not see my own example as an indictment of polyamory, any more than any other breakup is an indictment of monogamy.

Part Two

Polyamorous Families with Children

5

CHILDREN IN POLY FAMILIES

Children's experiences depended in large part on their ages. Overall, though, the children seemed remarkably articulate, intelligent, self-confident, and well adjusted. While they dealt with the usual issues of childhood—difficulty sharing toys, middle school social issues, awkwardness—the children in these families appeared to be thriving with the plentiful resources and adult attention their families provided. These findings mirror those of other studies that included children in polyamorous[1] or "group marriage"[2] families.

AGE DIFFERENCES

Although I only interviewed children five years old and older, I was able to ask parents about their very young children and observe very young children in poly families. Logan Tex, father of two small children, said of his seventeen-month-old son, Pip:

> He recognizes Amelia, our good friend who rents the other half of our duplex, but he doesn't see her as much as he sees our girlfriend Rhiannon. My mom and her partner come down all the time, and my dad, too. We also have friends we met in our homebirth class we spend a lot of time with, we've never had to hire a babysitter. Rhiannon or his grandmothers have probably spent the most time with him. Given how he reacts when people walk in the door he seems excited to see them, about eight or ten people he reacts to that way.

At about a year-and-a-half old, Pip responded positively to the adults who routinely spent time with him, regardless of their level of sexual involvement (or lack thereof) with his parents. Developmentally, children that small are not even aware of sexuality, much less socially developed enough to understand adult sexual relationships. As such, adults who were consistently present and available to meet the children's needs would blend in to a montage of loving caretakers indistinguishable (to the infant or toddler) on the basis of their relationships to each other, and important because of their relationship to the child.

When I was waiting to interview her older brother, I chatted with three-year-old ("and a half," she pointedly reminded me) Kassie while she and Vanessa (another preschooler visiting for a play date with Kassie) played on the living room floor. When I asked the girls what they were playing, Kassie explained that the figures laid out before her were going on a trip and described the figures as "Mommy, Daddy, Hercules [the family dog], my Dave, and Bessie [a plastic horse]." I asked her about "my Dave," whom I knew to be her parents' boyfriend, and she responded that "he comes on the fun." Then she gestured toward Vanessa and said, "She don't gots a Dave. She just gots a mommy and a daddy." It was clear from Kassie's story, her facial expression, and the sympathetic tone of her voice that she viewed Vanessa's lack of a Dave as a clear disadvantage. Kassie also did not question or problematize Dave's presence in her life; he was simply "my Dave," there to go "on the fun." Among the children old enough to respond, three distinct age groups stood out: young children (five to eight years old), tweens (nine to twelve years old), and teenagers (thirteen to seventeen years old).

Young Children

Children between five and eight years old often did not notice that their families were any different from other families, and instead they took their family form for granted. Like those in monogamous families, young children in poly families responded to their environments with a self-centeredness characteristic of their developmental stage. Young children tended to view the adults in their lives through the lens of what the adult did for or with the child, and they placed much less emphasis on how the adults were related to each other. Rather than mentally categorizing a parent's partner as *mom's boyfriend*, young kids in poly families were far more likely to think of that person as *willing to be dressed-up* or *bringer of ice cream*. As an important consequence, the presence or level of sexual interaction among the adults was simply not germane to these young children's experiences or conversations.

This became abundantly clear to me when I chatted with seven-year-old Marni Ballard and her five-year-old brother Milo. They lived in a rambling, ranch-style home in the Pacific Northwest with their extended family, composed of Hillary, their mother; Geoff, their father; Jake, Hillary's boyfriend; Barbara or Grammy, Hillary's mother; and Garth or Papa, Barbara's boyfriend. Hillary, Geoff, and Jake shared the upper portion of the house with Marni and Milo, and Garth and Barbara lived in the separate apartment that occupied the lower level of the large structure. As I sat at the dining room table with Marni and Milo and asked them about their relationships with Jake and their parents, they would occasionally look at me with confusion. They described their interactions with Jake, their mom, and dad, and during a conversation about who put them to bed, Marni asked me, "Why do you just keep asking us about them? Papa and Grammy read to us before bed and stuff, too."

Clearly, my focus on the *polyamorous* aspect of their family overlooked other parts of the family that were just as, or more, important to the children. What mattered to the children was that they had five loving and attentive adults caring for them, taking them places, picking them up from school, and putting them to bed at night. The children did not categorize this wealth of attention by the sexual relationships among the adults: It made no more difference to Marni and Milo that Jake was their mother's boyfriend than it did that Papa was Grammy's boyfriend because the children interacted with both Jake and Papa as trusted adults who cared for them. The children did not factor in the sexuality among the adults because it was simply not germane to their relationships with the adults. The smorgasbord of love was available to the children regardless of the adults' sexual relationships, or lack thereof.

Tweens

Children between nine and twelve years old, or "tweens," were more aware that their families were different from many of their friends' families, and they were increasingly aware of how the adults interacted with each other than were their younger compatriots. Like other kids their age, they knew the adults had sex and preferred to know as little about it as possible. They also knew that other families were frequently different from their own families, and that this information could sometimes be upsetting to adults. Children in this category began to actively think about how to explain their families at school, to their peers, and to other adults. As they realized their families were different from many of their peers, tweens asked their parents questions about the family and considered what they would tell their peers if and when someone else noticed.

Inevitably, some of their peers did notice the extra adults, and tweens in poly families had to explain their families far more often than their younger siblings. Adam and Michelle Hadaway began attending the same school when the Hadaway quad coalesced and Michelle's family came to live with Adam's family. I asked what Adam's peers thought when his family suddenly expanded.

> Elisabeth: If people at school ask what's up with your family, what do you tell them?
>
> Adam: This kid Lawrence, in my same grade, he'll be like, "How are you related?"
>
> Elisabeth: You?
>
> Adam: Me and Michelle, cause we are in the same grade. But we just don't say anything. They'll just keep on guessing, and they'll never get it right.
>
> Elisabeth: When you just don't say anything, how do you get away with that? Without responding at all?
>
> Adam: They just get so confused, they quit. It's only middle school.
>
> Elisabeth: I'm sorry I keep asking you about this, it's just hard for me to wrap my mind around that you don't have to offer some kind of explanation. Like, it's an unusual family, so when people ask you and

you just don't say anything, how is it that you can get away without offering any sort of explanation?

Adam: They'll just think they know what's going on and they stop asking. But they probably don't.

Elisabeth: So they kind of make things up themselves, and you don't correct them?

Adam: Exactly.

Adam and Michelle's peers noticed that there was something unusual about their families, but they were not quite able to figure out what was happening with the many siblings who suddenly began attending the same school. Even so, Adam did not see it as problematic, and indeed he seemed amused by his peers' confusion. Among peers with divorced and remarried parents, adopted children, and single parents, an addition or subtraction of siblings has many possible explanations and blends in to the social background of constantly shifting relationships among serial-monogamous families. In this case, Adam did not find his unconventional family problematic and was able to pass with ease as one of his many peers with more conventionally blended families, though as we shall see in chapter 9, some of his siblings had more problematic experiences managing that information with their extended family members.

Teenagers

Teenagers from thirteen to seventeen were generally establishing an increasing level of independence and an identity formed outside of their families, more invested in exploring their own social relationships and sexualities than were their younger brethren. This had a number of consequences, including the teens having to explain their families in more complex social settings and being less focused on their parental relationships as their own social relationships eclipse familial bonds in emotional urgency. Teens in poly families often consider whether they want to have poly relationships themselves, or if they would prefer monogamy—something I discuss in greater detail later in this chapter. Generally, the teens in the study were like other teens in that they were more involved in their own social lives than their parents' social lives. In an interview when she was fifteen years old, Kethry Wyss explained why her poly family was

> yeah, whatever, no big deal. I have my own stuff going on. I'm still swimming [competitively on a team], have a lot of friends, and we're really into anime and make costumes and go to cons and stuff. It is a big DIY [do it yourself] thing, so Mama helps us sew so my friends know her, it's not like I hide them or anything, I still love them, I'm just doing my own thing and not so much in their business. I can't wait to be able to drive! Then I can go to practice, whatever, don't have to wait to carpool and they don't have to come pick me up.

Kethry continued from there with a litany of the fun things she could do once she could drive herself. Her specialized social environment—a diverse magnet high school in the California Bay Area—contributed significantly to her ability to see her poly family as "no big deal" because many of her peers were adopted or had single, divorced, or gay parents and so her own multiple parents were unremarkable. In addition to being fully engaged in her own life and "not so much in their business" when it came to the adults, Kethry later explained how she felt she could trust her parents and talk to them about anything. She had both the emotional and social distance developmentally characteristic of teens busy establishing their own identities, but she also had the support of devoted parents she felt she could trust.

COMING OUT

As far as sexual minority families go, poly families are not nearly as visible or recognizable as lesbian or gay families, so these families were often able to exercise wide latitudes when deciding to come out or not.

Children Coming Out to Peers

For the most part, children did not have to deal with coming out to strangers, classmates, coaches, or teachers. The popularity of *serial monogamy*—a cycle of coupling monogamously/marriage, breaking up/ divorce, and coupling monogamously with someone else/remarriage—

in the United States makes it commonplace for children to have multiple parents. Now that stepparents are standard social fare, kids from poly families with several parental figures simply blend in. Unless poly family members intentionally highlight and explain their family structure, they are rarely called upon to justify their "extra" members.

If they choose to come out, children in poly families do so selectively, revealing family details only to those they know and trust, or those who ask politely in low-risk or need-to-know situations. Sebastian, a white high school student and Nash Majek's younger son, reported that he blended in among the varieties of families his peers inhabited.

Sebastian: No um surprisingly a lot of people in my school have like kind of like this situation with parents not really, not as far as I know not like polyamorous, but like parents issues.

Nash: Like divorced.

Sebastian: Yeah.

Elisabeth: So they'll have multiple parents like divorced and remarried?

Sebastian: Yeah, some people do.

Elisabeth: So do you feel like you're different from your peers?

Sebastian: No, not really, it's kind of normal to some people, if they don't have that happen to them because there are other people that have had it happen to them.

Elisabeth: It meaning? What's it?

Sebastian: Like just like the divorce issues or just, just parental issues . . .

Like many of his peers, the various adults in Sebastian's life blended in with his social surroundings, and he was rarely called upon to explain them.

In a sea of single parents, divorced, remarried, and cohabitating adults with children they bore or adopted, poly families may appear to be just another blended family. Their status as sexual minorities, however, presents different issues than their peers in (ostensibly) monogamous and heterosexual families. I asked Sebastian:

Elisabeth: Do you ever feel like you need to hide it from your peers or like you can't talk to them about it?

Sebastian: No, but I haven't told anybody about the polyamorous thing.

Elisabeth: How come?

Sebastian: Never really came about.

Elisabeth: If someone asked you about it, what would you say?

Sebastian: I would go ahead and tell—well it depends on the person. 'Cause there I know some, some kids are there at my school are like they have major Christian families or other beliefs that don't think it's OK to have multiple partners. I would only lie to them.

Elisabeth: Only lie to the Christians?

Sebastian: Yeah. Well, like that are strict about that. Some are flexible that they don't really mind that don't meddle with other people's business. But some are like . . .

Nash: Have you had a friend over when Morgan was there?

Sebastian: Um, I don't think so, not that I can recall.

Nash: I don't think so, but I know his brother Beck has.

Elisabeth: Do you know how that went with his brother?

Nash: Um, by all appearances . . . so this friend that um his brother has is one who has been a friend for some time and uh . . . you know knows that I am married to Marcy and has met her. Um . . . And so he saw you know Morgan at our house and that she was spending the night, and I think Beck told him that she was my girlfriend. And as far as I know he was completely oblivious.

Elisabeth: Mmmhmmm. How do you know Beck told him?

Nash: I think I heard him on the phone when we were discussing plans for his friend possibly coming over that um . . . I am pretty sure he used the term that "my dad's girlfriend was here" or that my dad was going to go do, go out, you know, I'm pretty sure he used the word *girlfriend*.

Elisabeth: Did your son say anything about the way his friend reacted?

Sebastian: Um . . . this certain friend, he has parents who are divorced, so he would probably be like "okay." He really wouldn't care.

Nash: That is exactly how he stated it. Okay, whatever.

It was clear from this exchange that Sebastian and most likely Beck did not care about their father's polyamorous relationship, rarely had to think about what to say or how to hide the information, and did not feel excluded from their peer groups.

Characteristic of this lack of tension around coming out, Zane Lupine—a seventeen-year-old white male high school student—said that he had never felt uncomfortable about being in a polyamorous family.

If a friend came over and both of my dads were there I would just tell them straight out, that's my other dad. If they were a little weirded out, I didn't take it as anything. I was never ashamed about it or never thought it was weird. I never really had to come out about it. If someone wanted to ask, they could ask but I wasn't going to just like . . . it wasn't something I had to announce, because it wasn't something embarrassing for me that I was trying to hide. If someone wants to know they can know, but I'm not going to go screaming about it. It's just not what I do about anything in my life really. I just don't ever talk about that kind of stuff that much. I guess if it came up, but it doesn't come up that much. I just never think to bring it up because it's normal to me. . . . It just obviously was not a big deal.

While the Lupine family originally lived in a small town in the Midwest, they had moved to a more liberal college town near a larger city when Zane was a child, so he was attending a fairly large, liberal, and diverse (for the area) public high school in an upper-middle-class, suburban neighborhood.

Other children, however, had far more difficulty dealing with their polyamorous family identities. Cole Cypress, a fifteen-year-old white male high school student, related how tremendously awkward and uncomfortable he felt when deciding to disclose his family formation to peers at school.

> Cole: It's always been very hard to explain to my friends at school, especially since I go to a private school. And I just feel, my friends would just be like, who's that person that's picking you up? And I'll just be like, that's Bettina, my mom and dad's girlfriend. It's kinda hard when you say that. . . . And then for a while I would do "family friends" and then when I got into about eighth grade they finally realized that I had a lot of people coming to pick me up and it was kind of weird to have so many family friends and some of the closer people, the people that were closer to me, I started explaining it in the best way I could. And it was really hard, but after they knew it was kind of a load off, you know. It's kind of weird to live with a secret, something you can't tell any of your friends cause they wouldn't understand.
>
> Elisabeth: So when you said it was kind of hard . . . telling them was hard?
>
> Cole: Yeah.
>
> Elisabeth: Or keeping it a secret was hard?
>
> Cole: Both. And trying to fit in, especially since I was not one of those kids that was the cool kid. I was never popular, I never had a lot of friends, especially in my earlier years. It was only in eighth grade when I think I actually made any real type of friends. But yeah, it was hard because, like when Bettina first came to pick me up at school one day I just tried to kind of explain how she wasn't my new mom but she was like my dad's girlfriend or something and you know it was just kinda weird.

In this case, Cole's discomfort with revealing his unconventional family life magnified his shyness and difficulty making friends. For Cole and other members of poly families, polyamorous relationships can magnify preexisting personal and relational issues. The same way a piece of metal will break along a fault line when stressed, the intensity and complexity of poly relationships place stress on issues in relationships that already existed but might not have come to a head in the same way if the relationship or family were monogamous. Long-term polys attempt to face these challenges head-on, using them as opportunities for growth or to explore personal boundaries. Others find that the added stress makes the issues too disadvantageous to pursue and decide that a polyamorous relationship form is not for them.

Other researchers have also reached similar conclusions in their research. In her book *Border Sexualities, Border Families in Schools*, Dr. Maria Pallotta-Chiarolli found that polyamorous and bisexual families in Australia used three primary strategies to present their unconventional families at school: 1) *passing* as a conventional family by staying quiet about their differences and attempting to blend in; 2) *bordering* regular and unconventional society by straddling both worlds, moving between them as needed or desired (what Pallotta-Chiarolli calls a *mestizaje*);[3] or 3) *polluting* by infiltrating a formerly monogamous social setting and openly displaying their social unconformity.[4] Many of these families used different strategies at different times, or blended characteristics of each as the situation demanded. Sebastian Majek had no problem passing as a member of a conventional family, and Adam Hadaway easily navigated the border, even in the face of his peers' scrutiny, simply by evading their questions. While Adam and Sebastian—both attendees at suburban public high schools—managed these interactions with ease, Cole Cypress's smaller and more tightly knit private school intensified peer surveillance and made it more difficult for him to pass. Cole's attempt to border met with mixed results, and he was pushed somewhat unwillingly into the role of polluter. In chapter 9 I return to Pallotta-Chiarolli's concept of polluting when I discuss respondents' strategies for dealing with stigma.

Parents Coming Out to Children

Polyamorous parents came out to their children in a variety of ways, and at a variety of points in their relationships, depending on the age of the children, the past and current familial configurations, and factors external to the family. Sometimes parents come out at different times or in different ways to their various children, tailoring the timing and information to the children's needs and the family situation.

If a child is born into a polyamorous family, parents will often wait until the children ask something about the family and then give age-appropriate information in direct response to a request. Marcus, the middle child in the Amore family, estimated that he was seven or eight years old when he first asked his parents, Louise and Max, about their family.

> They never paraded their partners around in front of us. They never tried to hide it, but they never threw it in our faces. They kept it private. . . . We were in the car and they were talking about their other partners, and . . . [when] I questioned them on this, they simply said they were polyamorous. I don't remember the exact words, but it was all simple enough. They were patient enough and helped me to understand it.

In contrast, Louise came out as polyamorous directly to Marcus's older brother Dave because, as Dave bluntly put it, "I was an eavesdropper." He continued:

> Dave: She told me when I got a little bit older. I think it was around ten or eleven, not real sure. I think part of the reason she told me is because, when I was that age I was an eavesdropper. I could be down in the basement and I could hear what's going on, on the top floor.
>
> Elisabeth: How so?
>
> Dave: I just have really good hearing. The vents sometimes helped, depending on which room you're trying to hear. But I just have really good hearing. I also have really good sight. I can read lips. Things like that help.
>
> Elisabeth: So when she talked to you about it, what did she say?

Dave: I don't know. I'm not really sure. She basically explained the situation. She cares for this person; this person . . . I'm like, "Okay, whatever makes you happy."

Elisabeth: It sounds like you weren't freaked out about that.

Dave: Yeah, I wasn't freaked out. I'm like, whatever. I'm gonna go play with my toys and go hang out with my friend Matt. Which I'm still friends with . . . I'm like whatever makes you happy. I'm going to go do something now. Go play with my friends. It didn't really occur to me that it was that unusual, I guess.

At the time, Dave did not see it as unusual and in fact wondered a little why his mother was "making kind of a big deal out of it." It was normal life for Dave and his siblings, so their poly family did not require much explanation.

When people who are already parents become polyamorous, they are more likely to have a coming-out conversation with their tween or teen children. Sebastian reported that his parents came out to him in a conversation much like the one Dave's parents had with him:

Um, it kind of took me by surprise I guess. They just kind of called me into the room and they just kind of told me. Like, we both love other people, and I was just like, okay. So it wasn't . . . it kind of surprised me because I hadn't really thought about it before. But I heard some . . . there were some clues about it, I forgot what, but . . . I just kind of . . . it took me by surprise, I just deal with it. I can't really care after a while.

Other tweens and teens knew something was going on but avoided the subject, did not want to know any more about it, and refused to discuss it. Elise Heartland said that

they didn't really sit us down and have a big talk or anything. We were sitting around watching TV and something came on, some gay guy or something, and I joked around, something about Sven, and I was like, well, are you bi? And he didn't really say anything so then I was like, it's fine, I don't really need to know. And something about Adam came up and it was like, I gotta go, I gotta get outta here. I need to go to my room. Really, it's just like, even knowing you guys have sex is enough, but I don't need to know anything beyond that, so why would I go out of my way to ask more about something I don't want to know anyway?

Much like children in monogamous, blended, or single-parent homes, children in poly families generally preferred not to know about their parents' sex lives.

SEXUALITY

Although it is somewhat awkward to point it out, any study of children in sexual minority families has to address the *sexual* aspect of the sexual minority (as if heterosexuality is not a form of sexuality as well, or as if most sexual abuse and incest didn't happen in heterosexual families). But the point became clear the more I spoke to poly families: none of my respondents had sex with or in front of their children. None of the children reported it, and none of the adults mentioned it either. One significant exception is a child who was molested by a parent's partner, which I discuss in far greater depth in chapter 7. I looked long and hard for the families with difficulties like custody suits in which children were most likely to be at risk, and found very few. Like in any family study, those who are molesting their children are far less likely to volunteer for research than are families who feel they have nothing to hide. Additionally, members of stigmatized groups often feel compelled to present the most positive image possible of their families in order to forestall any potential critique of poor or inappropriate care—something Pallotta-Chiarolli terms "passing as perfect"[5] and saw in her own study.

Children's Awareness of Parental Sexuality

It is not that these families were perfect, it is just that they were well within the range of usual experience and difficulties present in average family lives. When I asked adults about how they interacted in front of the children, they reported showing affection in an appropriate manner publicly and saving actively sexual interactions for the bedroom. I did not ask children explicitly about their parents' sexual interactions (focusing instead on the family's social interactions as a unit), but children would volunteer statements like Nolan Hadaway's, when he said: "I see them kiss and hug but nothing more mushy than that. Once I saw Pops swat Mom on the rear and she got him with the dishtowel, you know, like PG, and not even PG-13."[6]

Children reported being aware that their parents had sex but not wanting to think about it or talk much about it at all. In a tandem interview, best friends Heather Majek and Alice Heartland (both thirteen years old at the time, girls who attended the same middle school) each relayed their experiences growing up in a poly family. When I asked about their parents' public displays of affection, each made a face and gagging noises:

Alice: Well, they usually, let's just say that I know what they are going to do, once they send me downstairs.

Heather: Mine doesn't. They usually go upstairs, into their room, like they are "watching movies" (air quotes).

Alice: They'll be like, it's 9 o'clock, your bedtime. And I'm happy to leave! Cause I don't wanna be there watching them. Weird! Even though they don't just do it right there, in front of your face. . . . It's like awk-ward! Yeah. Because I never thought about Adam or Richie in that way. I don't like to think about it. I don't want to think about it. Yeah, it's just not . . . It's kind of weird. "Oh, there's my friend Adam up there. Wonder what they're doing." You know. It's really awkward.

Heather: I mostly see them kiss hello or goodbye, it's not like if we go to a movie they're making out or anything.

Alice: It wasn't as awkward as when I was younger. I didn't even know at all what they were doing. I was like, "Oh they just want me to go to bed. Whatever." It was no big deal at all. But now I understand and it's weird, but they love each other so I don't care.

While Alice and Heather were aware that their parents had sex and were fairly grossed out by it, the children were neither exposed to nor traumatized by it.

Elise Heartland's experience contrasted with her younger sister Alice's. Piqued by curiosity about Adam (Sven and Shelly's—Elise's parents—boyfriend) and unbeknownst to Elise, after high school one day some inquisitive friends had invaded Shelly and Sven's privacy while they were hanging out at Elise's house and discovered information regarding their sex lives. In an interview with Shelly and Sven, Elise reported:

> You guys don't know this but I got a lot of shit about Adam, I mean a lot. Because my friends all knew. They knew before I did.
>
> Sven: Really?
>
> Elise: They figured it out before I did. I was just like, he's over a lot, he's their good friend, they have friends over all the time. And it was finally like Jared, one of my good friends now but he was kind of an ass at the time, was like, "You know they do it—Svennie and little Adammie are getting it on." And I was just like whatever, you guys don't know what you're talking about. And my friends would spend the night and Adam would be like, "Suzanne, do you need a ride home or something?" and she would be like, he would give my friends rides home and it wasn't a big deal. We were in high school, we just laughed about it. And it wasn't a big deal. My excuse was always just, my parents are freaks you know, no big deal. My friends liked you guys up until the end of junior year and I would have people over and I remember one time it was like Jackie, Brad, and Jared went upstairs and found a bunch of stuff and it was like, oh shit.
>
> Elisabeth: A bunch of stuff like what?
>
> Sven: Porn.
>
> Elise: Sex toys. Yeah (hands clapping, laughing). So I got in trouble for that and I didn't even tell them to do that. Because I didn't even know that they did that. And they were just giving me so much shit about Adam and about them and I felt like I was always needed to hard-core defend them [Shelly and Sven], or I had no association with them, like they are freaks, they do what they want. I couldn't like be one or the other. I couldn't be accepting of it, either way,

because people are really closed-minded in high school. But now like when I see Jared or talk to my other friend online, if they say something I would just be like yeah, whatever.

Elise Heartland found her peers' awareness of her parents' sexuality alternately painful and tedious, a source of teasing even though her friends actually liked her parents. Even so, she was able to navigate her peers' ribbing and retain relationships with her friends over time. While initially Elise tried doggedly to pass as a member of a "normal" family— even to herself—her friends' discovery of her parents' collection of sex toys and pornography destroyed that fiction forever and forced Elise to transition to a new phase Pallotta-Chiarolli would call *bordering*, or managing her friends' knowledge of her family's unconformity in a monogamous social environment. Eventually Elise rebelled against what she saw as her friend's "asshole streak" and "closed-mindedness" and became what Pallotta-Chiarolli would see as a polluter, challenging the assumed dichotomous nature of families and her friends' short-sightedness. In fact, Elise asserted that polyamory had become a litmus test in her life, to some degree:

> If people can't deal with it, then I don't want to hang out with them anyway. I just can't get along with people so closed-minded, I don't wanna waste my time with assholes. Sometimes if I'm not sure about somebody I'll ask a question about gay marriage or something, or *Will and Grace*.[7] And if they're weird about that, I don't even bother with them. I don't need to be around anybody I have to hide my family from or I can't be myself around.

Generally, poly parents kept their sexuality private, and when the children did become aware of it, everyone involved actively sought to shield the kids from any specific knowledge of what went on behind closed doors.

Children's Ideas about Their Own Sexualities

Children's ideas about their own sexuality and future or current relationships varied primarily by age. Young children had no concept and did not tend to focus on or even understand sexuality. I did observe some play among young children, and I noticed on more than one occasion that when they would play family or house, they had a very wide interpretation of marriage that incorporated partners of the same gender or groups. It appeared to me that the normalcy of the poly family had permeated to the level of preschoolers' play. Tweens were aware of sexuality and felt varying degrees of comfort discussing it, from red-faced refusal and stuttering or simply confusion, to eloquent monologues about the pros and cons of polyamory and monogamy. Some teens had more definite opinions regarding their current and potential future relationships. For instance, teens such as Elise Heartland were certain they would not become polyamorous in the future. In response to my question about her thoughts regarding polyamory as a possibility for her, Elise responded:

> Would I ever be poly? Nooo-oooo, no way. I need way too much attention for that. I want to be the center of his attention, you know? Not sharing him with other girls. I watched my mom share Sven's attention for all of these years and it looked so hard sometimes. No, I want someone all to myself. Definitely not going to be poly.

Like her sister Elise, Alice Heartland thought it highly unlikely that she would establish a polyamorous relationship.

> Elisabeth: When you look forward into your life, do you see yourself being monogamous, polyamorous, how if at all do you see yourself?
>
> Alice: Just one person.
>
> Elisabeth: How come?
>
> Alice: I don't know. I think there would be jealousy. Like I'm going out with my other boyfriend today. I don't think that would make anybody really happy. So I think that's just why I'd prefer to stick with one person. I think there would be jealousy between, like well why aren't you going out to dinner with me, you know?
>
> Elisabeth: So you imagine other partners being jealous of your partners. Do you imagine yourself being jealous of other people?
>
> Alice: Yeah.

Elisabeth: You're concerned about your own jealousy and their jealousy.

Alice: Yeah.

Elisabeth: So anything else besides jealousy make you wanna steer clear of—

Alice: Not really. Well you like who you like, there's not really anything you can do about it. If it happens it happens I guess, but I don't really think so.

Elisabeth: You're not gonna look for it on purpose?

Alice: Yeah, I'm probably just gonna stick with one person for any relationships.

While Alice feared the high likelihood of jealousy within a poly relationship, she remained open to the potential for someone she liked to draw her into a poly relationship.

Heather Majek did not actively reject polyamory, but rather she simply accepted monogamy as the default that guided her relationships.

Elisabeth: Okay, so did you say, Heather, on your demographic form—You're dating, you cutie.

Heather: Hee.

Elisabeth: You, how's that going?

Heather: Good.

Elisabeth: How long have you been dating? Your form said you are heterosexual, so probably a dude, a boy?

Heather: "A dude." (laughs)

Elisabeth: A dude. How's it going?

Heather: Um, good I guess.

Elisabeth: Just the one dude?

Heather: Yeah. I don't cheat.

Elisabeth: You don't cheat. So seeing more than one dude would be cheating?

Heather: Yeah.

Elisabeth: How come?

Heather: I don't know.

Elisabeth: That's just the way it is.

Heather: Yeah.

Elisabeth: Okay. Did you and the dude talk about it?

Heather: Hmm?

Elisabeth: Like, decide that you were just going to see each other. Or was it just assumed?

Heather: It's just what everybody does, in junior high I guess.

Rather than making an explicit choice to be monogamous, Heather Majek fell into the general cultural trope of monogamy by default. Her parents' polyamorous relationship did not exert enough sway over her thought process to supersede the weight of the monogamous culture at large or the more immediate social circle of her junior high school. Clark and Morgan Majek refrained from proselytizing to their children and did not encourage them to become polyamorous, and in the absence of that pressure Heather had chosen the path of least cultural resistance at thirteen years old, with no serious thought to what she might want from a future relationship or family.

Zane Lupine took a flexible approach to his own potential to be polyamorous or not. When explaining why he was in a monogamous relationship with his girlfriend of two years, Ekaterina, Zane reported:

Zane: I just like the one that I'm with, so I don't really need anyone else. I guess if I felt that I needed more variety then I'd just be open about it and get more variety. But I don't feel that need for it or want it.

Elisabeth: Did you and Ekaterina ever talk about OK, are we going to be polyamorous, or are we going to be monogamous?

Zane: No, it's kind of like the classic—it's ninth grade so it was less mature I guess. "Would you go out with me?" kind of thing. It started where it was just that. We were boyfriend and girlfriend. Neither of us were expecting it to last very long—like most high school relationships, you know. But then it just did and we became like best friends. We've been together for like two years. There's never been a question of what we are, it's just kind of happened.

Elisabeth: And is she the same age as you, seventeen now? So she was fifteen when you got together, you were both fifteen? And now you're both seventeen?

Zane: Yeah.

Elisabeth: Do you have an agreement to be monogamous with each other?

Zane: Yeah, because if we cheated on each other it would probably be over I guess. We'd probably still be best friends, but we wouldn't have the relationship as boyfriend/girlfriend.

Elisabeth: How come?

Zane: I don't know, I haven't ever really looked at it any other way. I don't think she has either. That's just kind of how it started and how its been going.

Elisabeth: You don't have to discuss the rules, you just know?

Zane: Yeah, that's kind of how it is.

Elisabeth: Have you ever talked about potentially being polyamorous in the future?

Zane: No, I've never even thought of that. I don't really think too much about the future. That's I think, kind of a bad thing to do. I don't want to focus too much on the future, and just kind of keep going with it. I don't know, maybe sometime it will come up. Maybe if we keep on after high school, more stuff will be brought up, I don't know. I just know I don't get bored with her, that's why she's my best friend. I can always hang out with her, that's the reason it has lasted so long. I haven't gotten sick of her, she's always new to me. We always have something to talk about.

Zane was not interested in pursuing polyamory himself, at least at the moment, and he was not eager to make plans for the future. True to his mother Melody's Buddhist influences, Zane focused on staying in the moment and being open to what comes. True to society's influence, he automatically adopted social standards of monogamy that influenced so effortlessly that he and Ekaterina did not even need to discuss rules structuring their relationship.

Alternately, some people raised in poly families felt that monogamy would be far too stifling and they would definitely construct their own poly families. At fifteen years old, Marcus Amore had not established any serious romantic relationships, but he foresaw himself most likely being in a polyamorous relationship once he began dating:

I seriously want to try for polyamory. I have never really had issues of jealousy myself, however, not being in anything that I could consider a true romantic relationship, I'm not sure how jealousy would relate to that for me. . . . It has to do with freedom. I don't like the idea of restricting myself to a single relationship and I don't want to bind her to a single relationship. I know that much for certain. If I did have issues with jealousy and could not be in a poly relationship, then I could not allow our relationship to continue because I would not want to restrict her in that way.

Marcus's older brother Dave wasn't certain he would always be poly-amorous, but he felt more comfortable in a poly relationship than in a monogamous relationship. Discussing his two close female friends Annabeth and Kari, Dave described how they ended up in a polyamorous quad with Kari's boyfriend Kaden.

> Dave: Yes. I was in love with both of them. At first, it was really challenging. I wasn't sure quite what to do about it. Me, Kari, Kaden and Annabeth all sat down and talked about it. We ended up having a quad relationship. Annabeth dated me and Kaden, and I dated Annabeth and Kari.
>
> Elisabeth: And Kaden dated both Kari and Annabeth as well?
>
> Dave: Yes.
>
> Elisabeth: How'd that go?
>
> Dave: It was actually really nice for the first few months. One of the challenges that went wrong in that relationship, aside from the fact that we were all still young and all still into high school drama and bullshit—
>
> Elisabeth: Young meaning like seventeen?
>
> Dave: This was a year or two ago.
>
> Elisabeth: So seventeen-ish.
>
> Dave: Yeah, I was actually seventeen about to turn eighteen that summer. Two years ago, then. That went really well. One of the problems was, I didn't establish any boundaries. That ended up hurting the relationship, as well as a number of other things.
>
> Elisabeth: How did the lack of boundaries hurt the relationship?
>
> Dave: One of the things that I didn't know at the time, when I first went into the relationship is, I don't have a problem being polyamor-ous . . . The only time I really have a problem is when I have jealousy come up and it's very hard for me to deal with, is when I'm not being

distracted by work or by being with one of my partners. So I'm sitting at home going ughn! (Brooding sound) And just steaming.

Elisabeth: So you were saying that lack of boundaries and jealousy . . .

Dave: Yes. I didn't establish any boundaries. One of the things I learned later on is that, while I don't mind someone dating someone else that I'm dating, it does bother me if I don't have anything else to do or distract me. Whether it's work or anything else. That's something that's bothered me. I've gotten better about it, but at that time it was something that was really bad for me. That was probably just one of many things. It just started a chain of events and caused the relationship to fall apart.

Even though the relationship was imperfect and lasted no longer than many other high school romances, Dave felt that it had been a good thing for him and for the other quad members. They all continued to be friends, and Annabeth and Kari continued a sexual relationship after breaking up with both Dave and Kaden at different times.

It came as no surprise that the teens in polyamorous families were often undecided about their potential future sexual partners or relationship styles. None of them reported feeling pressured to become polyamorous in the future or feeling that their choices were constrained. Even more striking, these teen's automatic acceptance of monogamy indicated the social strength of that convention, even among those raised in families that practiced nonmonogamy.

WHO DO CHILDREN SEE AS PARENTS?

Four primary factors contributed to whether or not children saw adults as parents or not. The first and most obvious was a biological connection: all of the children know who their biological parents are. In her book *Pregnancy and Polyamory*,[8] Jessica Burde describes some polyamorous families who either intentionally avoid knowing the biological parentage or accidentally become pregnant in a situation where multiple men might be the biological father, so there are clearly a number of ways to approach childbearing in polyamorous families. The second most likely factor influencing a child's likelihood to view someone as a parent is the child's age at the relationship onset: the younger the child, the more likely the adult will move into a parental category in that child's mind. Third, children are more likely to see adults who share a living space with them as parental figures, so cohabitational partners are more likely to become parental figures than are noncohabitational partners. Fourth, it depends in large part on how long the person has been around the child and how much time they spend together. Those children who know an adult for many years and/or regularly interact with an adult over time are more likely to view that person as a parental figure than they are a relative newcomer or someone who is present infrequently.

Children reported viewing the adults in their lives as akin to aunts/ uncles, older siblings, or friends far more often than they thought of them as parents. In a conversation with me and her parents Shelly and Sven Heartland, Elise explained that she did not see Adam—Shelly and Sven's former boyfriend—as a father figure.

> Elise: No, not at all. But he was a really cool guy and a great friend and stuff. But since he was so young and I felt like a lot of the time he was more on my level than on their level or something . . .
>
> Shelly: But I think Alice viewed him as more of a parental figure because she was so young.
>
> Sven: She even called him daddy number two.
>
> Shelly: She would listen to him like a parent, where Elise, she was too old for that.
>
> Elise: And Adam came along when I was like sixteen, or fifteen, or something, so first of all it was like, "What is going on here?" Like, this is a little weird. But when I got used to it, it was like fine and stuff.

For Elise and many older children, parents' partners were often trusted adults the young people could rely upon for advice, attention, and assistance, but the partners were not often parental figures themselves.

In contrast, Kethry Wyss views all of the Wyss quad members as parents. Born into a poly family and cared for by the entire quad for fourteen years, Kethry did not distinguish between her biological parents and her social parents: they were all simply parents to her. This assumption created such a clear substratum in how she spoke about her parents that I do not have a single quote exemplifying her attitude toward her parents *as* parents per se. Kethry's silence on the topic of who counted as a "real" parent and her discussion of all four Wyss adults as her parents clearly indicated that she viewed them all as parental figures, regardless of biological or legal connection. They had all lived with and cared for her from infancy, and that is what made them parents.

Marni and Milo Ballard held a fairly amorphous view of the many adults in their lives who cared for them. Rather than distinguishing strongly between adult roles, the children seemed comfortable with adults who could occupy numerous roles. Marni reported that her parents' partner Jake was like a papa—the term Marni and Milo use for their grandfather—or a nanny, sometimes like an uncle.

> Marni: Once at dinner I asked what are we having for dinner? And he [Jake] said slugs!
>
> Elisabeth: So he jokes with you?
>
> Marni: Yeah. He is like a papa only funner. Or a nanny.
>
> Elisabeth: What makes him like a papa or a nanny?
>
> Marni: Because a nanny stays with children all the time and plays with them, and is like a parent only parents who can't control their kids [adults laughing in background], they're the nanny that comes to play with them . . . A papa is funny, I have a papa downstairs too. Jake is like an uncle but he's like a papa and like a nanny . . . Papa and Grammy live downstairs. Grammy kisses me and cuddles with me a lot, gives me gumball things . . . and Auntie Stacia comes to pick us up from school and sometimes she brings us treats.

The list of important adults in Marni and Milo's lives included people who loved and spent time with them, regardless of their biological or legal connections to the children or the other adults. In fact, their own family of origin was complex enough that their polyamorous family members simply blended in with the other chosen kinship relationships around them. Milo described his Papa this way:

> Papa is not really Mommy's dad. Grammy actually married a different grandpa, another grandpa, we have two grandpas, and Grammy married Grandpa instead of Papa and Grandpa is actually Mommy's dad. But we like to think that Papa is Mommy's dad. Even though he wasn't the daddy that made her, he helped her grow up.

With such a flexible understanding of parentage already, Jake's quasi-parental/uncle/papa/nanny relationship made complete sense to Milo and Marni.

Although most of the children I interviewed did not usually see their parents' partners as parental figures themselves, they did often see them as family members nonetheless. Marcus Amore reflected on his mother's partner Valentino:

> I guess for me, Val is most comparable to an uncle. I certainly don't see him as my father. Despite my real father's jokes about that, I never will. He is an adult male figure that I can look up to, but he is not my father and he has never tried to be. He has tried to be my friend and a member of my family, but never has he tried to replace anyone.

Expanding on what made Valentino a member of his family, Marcus said:

> It is a matter of attachment. He is very important to all of us; we all love him. He cares a great deal about us. We talk. If we need something, we can go to him about it. He'll help us when he can. That's what makes family, people you can count on. I consider my friends more than just that; I consider them my family. So in this respect, another advantage to being in a poly family is how I can view things as a result of this. You could say I have a very large, extended family, and I love that. I have many people I can talk to and connect to and go to for help. Generally I do not need to look beyond my own household for that, but if I ever do, there they are.

Like Marcus, other kids in poly families also had significantly expanded definitions of family that went beyond the scope of traditional biolegal definitions and included what scholars have usually termed *chosen kin*.

Speaking with me a few months after he moved across several states to live with Louise, Valentino agreed that he was emotionally close to Louise's children but did not see himself as their father.

> Elisabeth: Have you taken on a parental role with Louise's children?
>
> Valentino: Yes and no. I've developed a friendship with her children, who are just great people. Her sons and I play online games together, we go head to head against each other, that kind of thing. Her daughter's great, she and I have private chats sometimes where she confides in me a few things, and that's been nice. So probably just in the beginning, not too in-depth yet. I guess right now you can call it just more establishing a friendship with her [Louise's] family.
>
> Elisabeth: So I'm interpreting you to say that it's gone pretty smoothly—is that true?
>
> Valentino: Yeah.
>
> Elisabeth: Have you and Louise discussed any kind of shared responsibility for the children?
>
> Valentino: We've discussed that we need to discuss it [laughing]. Right now my role, until there is a full-blown family meeting, is that these are her children. This is her house. These are their rules. My involvement with the children as far as traditional guidance—I always leave that up to Louise. The schoolwork is to be done, Louise is the one. I simply ask them, you know, how their schoolwork is coming along. Any permissions to be going out with certain friends, they always have to ask Louise. You know, I treat them with respect and we can be friendly, but when it comes to making decisions that is up to Louise; I am not their guardian. "Louise is your mother, go check with her."

I asked if it ever became frustrating not being able to enforce anything as a parent, and Valentino responded:

Yeah, sometimes. Like, Louise told Mina to clean up after the dog in the back yard, not a fun job. And it was a forest, she couldn't really see what she needed to pick up. I said, "Would you please excuse us?" I wanted to go over her head and enforce that, but I couldn't. They're her kids. Discipline and all that stuff, I couldn't do it. So I simply asked Mina, "Are you going to be able to do this or not?" She says, "Yeah, but . . ." and unfortunately I got a little perturbed to the point where I said, "Yes or no—are you really gonna do this?" "Well, no."—"Thank you for telling me." And so I went over her, I went ahead and just did it. It probably wasn't the best way, but I just needed to know . . . I told Louise about it later and she said she was going to go ahead and have a chat with the kids. That's why it's another thing we added to the list of what we need to talk about.

Like many other poly families, the Amores used family meetings and other smaller group discussions to navigate the complexities of multiple parents and children sharing a domicile. They also exemplified the propensity for both children and adults to assign parental status to only those partners who entered the family when the children were young and have continued interaction over time that usually included cohabitation. In the absence of those factors, children and adults in poly families constructed relationships with chosen kin more likely to take on roles like those of aunts, uncles, cousins, or friends.

6

ADULTS IN POLY FAMILIES

The families who participated in the development of this book, on the whole, felt satisfied with their family lives, and cast polyamory as having a positive impact on themselves and their children. This optimistic tone could result from the reality that poly families are good for the people who live in them, and that the people in these families generally have race and class privilege so their lives are just easier on those fronts than people who don't have those privileges. It could also result from a group that feels judged by conventional society trying to make their unconventional choices appear as positive as possible in order to defuse possible criticisms.[1] Overall, these families seemed to work quite well for the people who continued to live in them.

FAMILY FORMS

The most common form of poly family seems to be an open couple with children (two people in a long-term relationship who often live together and have additional sexual relationships) and their attendant constellation of kin, both biolegal and chosen. Open-couple families appear to identify as family for longer periods than do larger groupings, which are rarer and experience greater membership fluidity. Some have children from previous relationships, others have children from their poly familial unions, and still others remain child free/child less and identify themselves as members of poly families composed of adults. While some people actively seek poly relationships for years and consciously construct a chosen family, others become polyamorous by spontaneously forming a relationship first and then coming to identify later as polyamorous.

POLYAMOROUS FAMILY ISSUES

Polyamorous families experience a number of relationship issues, including relations with biolegal families, marriage and commitment, and divorce. Because they have such a tremendous amount in common with families of other sexual minorities, and especially lesbians, bisexuals, and gays, in this chapter I include them as a comparison group and term them *lesbigays*.

Relations with Biolegal Families

Relationships with biolegal family members varied dramatically, from close and loving to severely strained or estranged. Similar to families of people who come out as gay, some families reacted especially negatively at first and then became more accepting over time. At one end of the spectrum, some of my respondents were at ease being "out" with their families of origin regarding their polyamorous relationships. For example, Louise Amore was comfortable being candid with her mother, JP, because

> my mom is poly too. She doesn't call herself that, but she has been my whole life. She was very open about her sexuality and we talk about our sex lives together all the time. . . . She doesn't judge me for anything, she's one of my best friends!

Key polyamorous ideals like communication and honesty cultivated the sense of intimacy Louise perceived between herself and JP, whose ostensible status as a potential polyamorist herself further reinforced their bond. Louise and JP's comfort with being candid with each other mirrored that of lesbigays who were also at ease being candid about their sexual orientations with their families of origin.[2]

The Tree triad—composed of Bjorn, Gene, and Leah, all with PhDs and academic or high-level industrial jobs—found that relationships with their families of origin that had been slightly strained by the triad's inception as a family became warmer as all six of the parents came to view themselves as grandparents to the triad's son, Will. While none of the parents outright rejected any of the Tree triad members, some did express significant concern over their adult children's well-being and fear that the unconventional lifestyle would potentially harm them emotionally.

Initially, this sense of dismay was significantly heightened for the triad's parents when Leah became pregnant and the triad refused to disclose to anyone which of the men was the biological father. The Trees felt strongly that they were a single family, and that distinguishing between the two men to designate one of them as the "real" father was fundamentally against their relational orientation. This refusal to identify the biological father was initially frustrating to the grandparents, but once Will was born their collective level of acceptance rose. Tree family members reported the following:

> Gene: We each have parents and so they are all equal grandparents of Will. No one came out to visit [for the birth] because we did not want anyone out, we wanted to deal with the initial weeks on our own and then they could come. We have enough manpower and wanted to get ourselves established first. The mothers were relieved; it is the first grandson on both dad's sides, even though Leah's brother has a son so I guess it is not really their first, but even so everyone is super excited about him [Will]. A month ago we had all the grandparents to a house on the East Coast and spent the weekend trading Will around and playing tennis.

> Elisabeth: So all of the grandparents are cool with you now?

> Leah: Yeah, there is no animosity with each other or with us—they have gotten over all the weirdness, and having Will sealed the deal with me and Bjorn's mom. They were still a little tense when we told them, there was a five-second beat of oh, my, well, of course, congratulations. Now they are soooo into him and his mom emails me all the time.

Bjorn: We visit with each grandparent every three or four months, and we Skype all the time. We have been to the East Coast and they have come here, so all of the grandparents have been able to spend time with Will fairly regularly.

The fact that "the grandparents" became (at least ostensibly) more accepting of the Tree's unconventional family style once they had a child is due both to the triad's patience and willingness to endure parental disapproval and the irresistible power of an infant to coax a reluctant grandparent's adoration. This increase of acceptance after a sexual-minority family has a child mirrors other researchers' findings in studies of the families of gays and lesbians, who reported that their own parents often accepted them or their partners to a greater degree once they had a child.[3]

Even in the absence of an irresistible infant, some families accepted their polyamorous family members with open arms. When Megan Holstrom's father died her husband, Billy, prepared to go to the funeral with her. Megan's boyfriend Jack, who lived in a neighboring state, responded to the news of his beloved's father's death with instant action. Billy reported that

> Jack just would not stay home. He said, you need support and I am coming to the funeral, you can't stop me. So we told her [Megan's] mom and she said, "You love each other?" We said yeah. "He is good to you?" Yeah. "Then that's great, as long as you love each other it's fine with me." Jack went to the funeral and helped fold the flag, which I thought was a huge acceptance on the part of the family because they had never met him and accepted him right away as a part of the funeral party.

In this case, Megan's family accepted both Billy and Jack as her partners with no further scrutiny beyond investigating their emotional commitment to each other, even integrating Jack into the funeral party.

The Wyss family has experienced a wide range of acceptance and rejection from biolegal family members. Kiyowara Wyss's experience with her grandmother's eightieth birthday party was at the positive end of that spectrum. The party was a major event for Kiyowara's mother, Suka, and her extended family members who were in attendance from various states in the United States and Japan. It was also the first such

event the entire quad attended as a family unit. Because of their appearance as two heterosexual couples, the Wyss quad expected the true
nature of their relationships to remain unrecognized. Kiyowara reported that, during the party, she was

> focused on my grandmother's birthday. You know, I didn't feel a
> need to make a statement about "We're here together" or anything.
> And I couldn't believe that, my mom was up on stage thanking every-
> one for coming and she called us all up and she said, "I want to
> introduce you to my children" and that was it. Everybody knows that
> me and my sister are her only *biological* children, so some of them
> had no idea what she was talking about. But now we're all her kids
> and that was that! I was really touched, for her, you know, to do that,
> it really meant a lot.

Kiyowara thought that her mother's public acknowledgement of all the
spice as her children was Suka's way of recognizing the legitimacy of
Kiyowara's unions. Suka's public acceptance of the quad facilitated
friendly contact between herself and the quad, as well as their interactions with Suka and Kiyowara's extended family.

In the Wyss quad's case, Suka's acceptance waxed, waned, and ultimately proved to be firmly rooted in the quad's ostensible heterosexual
relationships. Over time Suka became quite ill and moved in with the
quad to recover from a hospitalization. She was in pain, bewildered, had
trouble breathing, and had to be monitored around the clock. Because
she was already Kethry's full-time parent at the time, Loretta agreed to
care for Suka as well. In an effort to manage the considerable caretaking demands, Loretta sought assistance from many state and federal
agencies and was scrupulously forthcoming with the various social
workers, home health aides, and assistants regarding the adults' polyamorous relationships. Suka, however, frequently tried to conceal the sexual relationship between Loretta and Kiyowara by telling the host of
personal and medical assistants that the two were sisters. Loretta sus-
pected that Suka's initial ostensible acceptance might have provided a
cover for her veiled discomfort and homophobia that emerged as her
flagging health became increasingly problematic. Like Suka, Kiyowara's
extended biolegal family was similarly ambivalent, happy to accept Loretta's role as a full-time caregiver and the Wyss family's continual
financial gifts (including purchasing two different homes for Suka), but

unwilling to grant the Wyss family recognition as genuine family members at Suka's funeral.

Similar to the Wyss family, the Southern triad had a spectrum of relationships with their biolegal families, from affable to horrid. Triad members were Earl, Tom, and Melinda, all in their early forties. Tom and Melinda were married for eleven years and had two children when they formed a triad with their longtime friend, Earl. Each member of the triad invited their parents to the commitment ceremony that marked their eventual coalescence as a family unit. Earl reported that his parents were "thrilled . . . they'd given up on ever having grandkids when I came out to them as gay, so to have two ready-made grandkids put them into grandparent heaven!" While Melinda's parents were accepting, they were notably less enthusiastic than Earl's. The most politically and religiously conservative of all the Southern triad's biolegal kin, Tom's parents not only rejected the triad's invitation to the ceremony, they then rebuffed further contact with that entire family (including their grandchildren).

Things changed, however, four years later when Tom's father was diagnosed with cancer. Tom's mother called him to let him know his father was in the hospital, and she said "life was too short to hold this kind of a grudge." His father consented to speak to Tom, and while he was happy to be "patching things up," Tom's parents' initial rejection still hurt. "Things can't ever be the same again once your parents have told you that you aren't their son anymore."

Some respondents came from complex families of origin, so their poly families were not particularly shocking to their biolegal and chosen kin. Logan Tex was characteristic of respondents who came from unconventional backgrounds and became polyamorous. Logan was in an open-couple relationship with his wife, Melina, and their girlfriend Rhiannon. At the time of the interview, Melina and Logan had two small children, an infant and a toddler named Pip less than two years apart. Logan's parents had split up when he was a child, so his family of origin included his mother, Jess, her wife, Paula, his father, Nick, and his wife, Erin—all of whom took parental roles to some degree in Logan's life—as well as a variety of siblings from several combinations of parents and their exes. When I asked him what his family of origin thought of his poly family, Logan replied:

My moms seem generally supportive of whatever I do. Paula, my biological mom's partner, feels Rhiannon might be trying to steal me away and doesn't like her in the middle of my family. Jess, my bio mom, is fairly distant with Rhiannon. It's hard to get a read on her. My dad seems to be envious that I can have the life I do—his wife does not like him being with other women, but I think he would [do so] happily if the relationship allowed for it.

The fact that Erin, Jess, and Paula all reacted slightly negatively to Rhiannon—a common reaction among mothers-in-law to their son's girlfriends who retain sexual ties to other partners—is ironically conventional, considering that Jess and Nick had raised their children in a decidedly unconventional lifestyle. Logan links his upbringing directly to his contemporary poly family:

I think my childhood heavily influenced how I am. But I am still figuring out how, exactly. I was raised, somehow, to not have much regard for traditional ways of doing things—divorce, gay parents, parents that still talked and were friends postdivorce all played in to that. I learned that relationships can evolve, which means that the risk of a romantic relationship is less, since you can keep something if the romance part goes . . . I was raised on a hippie commune and those adults are still my friends, not just people my parents knew. I liked that and would like to give that to my kids. One of the features of that is that is they have been friends for decades, which means committing to being friends. As far as romantic relationships go, it would be important to me to maintain friendships even if the romantic part ends.

For Logan, bonds outside of conventional marital life can be enduring and outlast divorce, supersede romance, and become lifelong commitments among friends—definitional of both chosen kinship and poly-affectivity. While his mothers allow for and themselves express wide social variation, they remain somewhat uncertain about their son's poly family. Logan himself has mixed feelings about conventional relationships himself, as we shall see in the next section.

Marriage and Commitment

People in same-sex relationships seem far more interested in attaining legalized same-sex marriage than do polyamorists, who appear to be significantly less personally or politically devoted to plural marriage.[4] My findings indicate that respondents do not mention marriage as a central concern, and when they do, some do so disparagingly. Those poly people who wish to marry can do so as pairs, and the tendency toward hetero and bisexuality among polys makes it possible for them to (ostensibly) meet requirements for heterosexuality. Because most of the people in this book are white and middle-class professionals, their race and class privileges offer some protection against discrimination,[5] making the rights associated with legal marriage less important for polys than they would be to others with fewer social privileges. Such access grants polys greater social maneuverability than those in recognizably same-sex relationships, a latitude that is reflected in polys' views of marriage. Some reject marriage as inherently flawed; others are married but do not see it as very important; and still others view marriage as profoundly important in shaping their relationship structures and interactions.

Commitment Ceremonies

Poly folks expressed a variety of views about marriage and commitment ceremonies. Like some lesbigay couples, polyamorists occasionally formalize their commitments with public ceremonies that acknowledge the group as a family unit. For some, ceremonially announcing that they are "fluid bonded" (a negotiated safer-sex agreement that allows people to share bodily fluids only with specific lovers who have been tested for STIs) signals their lasting pledge to their partners and communities at large. One trio of two women and a man who had dated for several years gleefully informed the attendees at their ceremony/party that marked their fluid bonding that "we are a family now!" Other polys choose alternative forms of union such as handfasting, a Pagan ritual in which people are ceremonially bound wrist to wrist with soft cord for three days and thereafter considered to be married.

Occasionally large and stable families like the Wysses deal with the lack of official recognition by creating corporations or trusts to manage taxes, child custody, medical power of attorney, inheritance, and joint property ownership. As scholars documenting lesbigay's attempts to secure similar legal rights find, such arrangements require extensive legal documentation in an attempt to address every foreseeable contingency, from the division of property in case of "divorce" to the assurance of continued custody of children if both biological parents die.[6] The high cost of this legal documentation makes this route almost impossible for anyone without significant financial resources for such extensive legal preparation.[7]

Marriage

Because many polys can legally marry as ostensibly monogamous, heterosexual couples, they have different relationships with marriage than do most lesbigays. While lesbigays may also choose to marry someone of another sex in a similarly ostensibly monogamous and heterosexual couple, it requires a far greater effort to maintain a closeted gay life than it would for polys with other-sex partners—a configuration that makes them socially recognizable as heterosexual couples with "close friends." This ability to remain closeted almost effortlessly is a resource many lesbigays cannot have, and so it functions as a form of (often misattributed) heterosexual privilege that provides a buffer against the effects of stigma against sexual nonconformists.

Few poly people talk about legal plural marriage at all, and even fewer identify it as an important goal. Some polys avoid or even ridicule monogamous marriage as an ill-conceived experiment. Joya Starr told me: "I think [marriage] is an institution, and that's fine if you want to be institutionalized." Others scorned people in monogamous marriages as "coasting" or "on automatic pilot." Thaddeus, a forty-one-year-old musician, cast marriage as detrimental to the health of relationships: "The thing that ruins their marriage was a piece of paper saying that they were married . . . There wasn't communication, that these were things that they certainly couldn't talk about because they felt stuck." Polyamory provides Joya and Thaddeus a vantage point from which to critique monogamous families and relationships, much like those who oppose same-sex marriage because they contest all marriage or advocate decoupling social benefits from relationship status.[8]

Like the majority of polyamorists who have participated in research, Joya and Thaddeus were both white, well educated, and middle class—with access to the privileges that allow them to focus on rebellion against the patriarchal norms of conventional families. Their socioeco-nomic status and cultural cache provide the kind of security that is scarce for lesbigay and/or working-class people. The larger and more diverse lesbigay community has a broader range of people, and the social privileges that attend legal marriage can be far more important to those who have few other privileges. The more scarce the privileges, the more precious each becomes. Mainstream polyamorists' myriad privileges allow them to downplay or forgo marriage in favor of rebel-lion precisely because they are so well endowed in other areas.

In some cases, legally married polys cast their marriages as inconse-quential. Phoenix and Zack, a white couple in their early sixties, date their relationship from its inception over thirty years ago, rather than the date of their actual legal marriage, which Phoenix sees as "pretty much just a piece of paper. We did it so he could get health insurance—at the courthouse." Many legally married polys mention it only in pass-ing and do not identify it as important in their interviews, but they are still able to avail themselves of its advantages and secure benefits that remain unavailable to their counterparts in same-sex relationships. This near-universal poly disinterest in legalizing multiple-partner marriage, or even investing heavily in conventional marriage, stands in sharp contrast to the significance many lesbigays accord same-sex marriage.

In rare instances, legal marriage plays a significant role in shaping partners' expectations of each other. For example, the Hadaway quad members had complex attitudes toward marriage. The quad is com-posed of two legally married couples and their ten children (five from each couple), with sexual relationships between the women and both men independently, but not between the men. Its members, all in their early forties, include: Gwenyth, a full-time homemaker; her legal hus-band, Mitch, a real-estate broker; Tammy, a part-time assistant to both Mitch and Gwenyth; and her legal husband, Phil, an electrician and technician. Each couple had been together for almost fifteen years when the women, both pregnant with their fifth child, met in an Inter-net parenting chat room and began an online relationship that was mostly friendship with, Tammy reported, an undercurrent of "strange intensity." After meeting in person with their spouses and eventually establishing "cross-coupled" sexual relationships between Gwenyth and Phil and Tammy and Mitch, the four decided that Phil and Tammy would move from their neighboring state to live near Mitch and Gwenyth. Shortly after arriving, Phil had a nervous breakdown, partially in response to the tremendous stress of working in the Gulf Coast region of the southern United States after hurricane Katrina had devastated New Orleans and the surrounding areas. Phil reported that "it had been coming for a long time," and Mitch opined that Phil was "finally able to let go once he knew there was someone else there to take care of his family." Tammy and Phil subsequently moved in with Mitch and Gwenyth, blending their households and nine of their children (Tammy and Phil's eldest daughter moved to her own apartment).

Tammy reported that Phil expected her to make him breakfast every day before he left for work—even though Gwenyth was already up getting the children ready for school—specifically because she was his wife and "that is the kind of thing a good wife does." Phil expressed dismay at what he saw as Tammy's waning devotion. "She used to do it when it was just her and me, but now that we live with them it's like she's not really my wife anymore. At least not the way she used to be." Similarly, Mitch considered his relationship with Gwenyth to be his priority, not only because they had been together for many years but also because they were married and thus should have primary allegiance to each other. Gwenyth reported feeling hurt by Phil's "fixation" on having Tammy do things for him. "I like spending that time with you and you don't appreciate it at all. It doesn't matter that we're not married, I still love you and can make your lunch!" She rejected legal marriage as the overriding relational structure, saying, "I don't recognize any primary-secondary, we're all on the same level," regardless of legal marital status. Even within this family, members did not necessarily agree on its terms. While this is possibly true of any marriage in which partners have differing views on the nature, function, or dynamics of their relationships, it can be even more pronounced in poly families. Retention of significant elements of monogamous or other patriarchal familial types can potentially impair adaptability, as the attempt to graft on elements of the previous form inevitably chafe against the new form. The quad experienced growing pains as they attempted to redefine their roles and relationships to each other, stretching their abilities to adapt to changing relational configurations and precipitating various crises and conflicts over mundane issues of daily life.

In contrast to the Hadaways who framed the issue as emotional and traditional connections between and among quad members, Logan Tex explicitly cited the privileges associated with marriage. When I asked him why he and Melina married, he responded:

> We decided to do it legally because it makes things a lot easier, legal things around the kids and being incapacitated and things like that. We were toying with the idea of writing our own nonmarriage contract with nothing about monogamy but we were lazy and took the easy route and just signed the state thing. But that means that there will on some level be some disparity with us and Rhiannon, even if she ends up living with us. I do not see us having another ceremony where we invite our friends and family to get married to Rhiannon. We have given a privilege to our own relationship over other relationships that is not particularly polyesque in a way, but on a philosophical level it is interesting that we chose this.

> Elisabeth: How does Rhiannon feel about this?

> Logan: Hard to say. She says she feels good about her connection to us as a family, but I think eventually she will want something deep with someone and thus her relationship with us will get a little more distant as she gives priority to someone else. Or she will become fully integrated with us. It's a weird position for her to be in and I can't imagine exactly what it's like.

Logan's assumption that, if their relationship progressed, Rhiannon would "end up living with us" and "become fully integrated with us" was based in couple privilege, something he acknowledged as "not particularly polyesque" but preferable to him and Melina. Well aware of Rhiannon's potential dissatisfaction, Logan knew that it might mean changing or losing his relationship with Rhiannon.

Logan and Rhiannon had begun dating roughly two years earlier when Melina was pregnant with Pip. Melina and Logan spent some time talking about their relationship and decided that if Logan was going to find a girlfriend:

> It was only going to get harder after we had the baby, so if I want a girlfriend I should find one now. Rhiannon is so much more of a girlfriend than I was really looking for. I was after someone to frolic with but she has become really important to us and much more integrated into our lives than we had anticipated. She and Melina

really clicked too. Melina was very pregnant when they first met and it was good for them to meet before the baby was born. Having the baby coming definitely put things on a timetable.

Even with the unexpected and slightly rushed beginning, over the next two years things had gone well with the Texes. Logan explained that "Rhiannon independently loves Pip, likes to spend time with him for the sake of spending time with him. We agree that it seems nice all around." While Rhiannon was subject to the disadvantages of being the secondary relationship, outside the protective circle delineated by couple privilege, she clearly got enough of her needs met in the relationship to stay in for at least two years, and possibly more.

DIVORCE

Polyamorists' various views on marriage parallel their similarly diverse relationships with divorce. Some of my respondents selected polyamory as an alternative to divorce, while others became poly subsequent to divorce from monogamous marriages. Still others divorced and retained sexual and/or cohabitational relationships with their "exes" after dissolving their legal unions. Most similar to lesbigay families, some members of disbanded polyamorous families did not have access to legal divorce.

Become Poly Instead of Divorcing

Some people transition to poly families rather than divorce. Typically this happens when one of the partners is discovered engaging in an adulterous affair or confesses a transgression to their spouse, and those involved choose extramarital relationships for both partners rather than divorce. Claire and Tim, a Mexican American woman and a white man both in their mid-thirties and married for nine years, decided to become polyamorous instead of divorcing when Claire learned of Tim's extramarital affair. Claire articulated feeling betrayed by Tim's initial deception but, while she did not want to be the "dupe who stays at home with the kids while he is out screwing around," she was not willing to end their relationship. Claire and Tim reconsidered the meaning and stability of their union, and they ultimately chose to open their relationship to outside lovers. Claire reported greater personal satisfaction and equality in her marriage since she has outside relationships as well, in part, she thought, because Tim no longer took her for granted as much. By agreeing to alter the definition of their relationship, Claire and Tim simultaneously reformed the power dynamic from a traditional familial structure rife with power imbalances to one that Claire thought "leveled the playing field." Poly families' flexibility permits them to adjust to shifting family circumstances, allowing families to outlast the crisis moment and reposition themselves to accommodate changes in structure and form, fostering an adaptable kinship network.

Polyamorous after a Divorce

Some people whose previous marriages ended because of cheating will begin a new relationship with the explicit intention of creating a polyamorous family. Sven Heartland's divorce resulted from his lying and hiding his sexual relationships with men from his now ex-wife, so Sven vowed to himself to be honest in future relationships to avoid making the same mistake again. When he met Shelly, Sven was forthright about his bisexuality from the beginning of their relationship. Initially shocked by Sven's suggestion to add a boyfriend to their family, Shelly eventually became more accepting of polyamory, though she remained somewhat dubious at times. "I never would have considered it before I met Sven, but I would rather be involved with these guys than have him taking so much energy and time away from the family to be with them."

For several years Shelly and Sven dated men with limited success. Ultimately they met and fell in love with Adam, a thirty-five-year-old white computer systems support provider with whom they established a triadic relationship. While the triad seemed to coexist peacefully for several years and all three members reported being happy together, the relationship eventually began to experience some difficulties. Shelly was more attracted to Adam than he was to her, and she occasionally felt some tension around this imbalance of desire. After almost four years together, Adam broke up with Shelly and Sven, who eventually began dating other men again. The flexibility of a poly family allowed Sven to be honest with Shelly and meet his need for sex with men while still retaining his familial connection with his wife and children. The frank dialogue characteristic of this and other poly families[9] similarly set the stage for Shelly to verbalize her needs and openly negotiate a safer-sex agreement.

Divorced but Still Lovers

Some polys divorced but continued their relationships much as they had prior to the divorce. Melody Lupine's triad was characteristic of this tendency to create new familial patterns. She had already had two children with Cristof, her legally wed husband, and she intentionally became pregnant with a third child when Quentin, her additional (extralegal) husband, expressed the desire for a child. Both Cristof and Quentin accompanied Melody in the delivery room when she gave birth to Zane, her second son. Though the triad specified paternity and expressed their intent to coparent, officials insisted on listing Cristof as the father on the birth certificate because state law stipulated that a married woman's husband is the legal father of any child she bears, regardless of evidence to the contrary. Melody said:

> We told everybody Quentin is the father. I'm married to Cristof, and Cristof's name had to be put on the birth certificate, legally, because we were married. Even though we said no, this is who is and this is who it isn't. And they were just like, we don't care. You're married, his name goes on. Quentin was outraged.

In order to clarify Quentin's relationship with his infant son and Melody's relationship with both men, the triad decided that a legal divorce was in order. Ironically, a social system designed to support families in this case actually encouraged divorce through its lack of flexibility. The Lupine triad's relational adaptability allowed them to outlast the legal marriage by negotiating a flexible arrangement to suit their kinship needs. Melody was optimistic about the impact the divorce had on the family, and she felt it set a good example for her children, who saw their parents remaining connected during a congenial divorce:

> They get to see that a divorce or break-up doesn't have to be this destructive, I hate this other person, I have to choose between mom and dad, I have to hear them arguing, they don't talk to each other.

> Children take on so much stress and trauma from divorce where
> parents pit one against the other. That didn't happen.

As society grows ever more complex and social changes we have
been experiencing for some time already continue, this ability to maintain friendly contact through changes in family life and structure is
becoming increasingly important. By deemphasizing biolegal connections and embracing a broader definition of family, both polys and
lesbigays demonstrate the resilience of polyaffectivity and chosen kinship.

Lack of Access to Legal Divorce

While divorce and its polyamorous proxy of separation exert a mixed
impact on polyamorous people and their children, the lack of access to
official divorce can sometimes be as difficult as a divorce itself. The
Mayfield quad, composed of Alicia, Ben, Monique, and Edward, all in
their late thirties or early forties at the time, was together for eleven
years before breaking up. Ben, Monique, and Edward had all been
employed during their term in the quad, but Alicia's back injury pre-
vented her from performing paid labor. Instead, she cared for their
home and Monique and Edward's biological children, who were five
and seven years old when the quad coalesced as a family. When the
quad disbanded, Alicia had no access to the usual recourses available to
women whose monogamous legal marriages end. Without legally recognized relationships to any other quad members except her soon-to-be-
ex husband, formalized access to the children she had cared for during
the last eleven years, or the legally recognized ability to seek the alimo-
ny traditionally awarded to homemakers who divorce a wage earner,
Alicia was in a difficult position indeed. Although legal protections
would not have shielded Alicia from the emotional impact of the family's dissolution, they would at least have allowed her visitation of the
children she reared and financial compensation for the years she spent
raising them and maintaining the household to facilitate the waged
work of her spice. Lack of official recognition of her polyamorous family
contributed to Alicia's personal and financial devastation. No marriage
means no divorce, and in many cases, no mediated negotiation of custody and property issues. Legal divorce is clearly far from perfect, but it

does provide some protections for nonbiological parents and homemakers that are unavailable to people in relationships that are not legally recognized. For both polyamorists and lesbigays who wish to marry or divorce, legal recognition remains a double-edged sword: it constrains the forms families are able to take, but the lack of those protections can be costly for those whose relationships are not recognized by the legal system.

WHEN IS A POLY RELATIONSHIP A SUCCESS? A FAILURE? OVER?

Although most families have divorced members in their kinship networks, conventional wisdom still defines a marriage or long-term relationship that ends in any other outcome besides death as a *failure*. Children of divorce are said to come from "broken homes"[10] and their parents have "failed marriages" that mark them as personal, relational, and often financial failures.[11] These cultural norms define "successful" relationships as monogamous and permanent in that the two people involved remain together at all costs. In this worldview, sexual fidelity is fundamental to the successful relationship and functions as both a cause and a symptom of relationship success.

Polyamorists, in contrast, define the ends of their relationships in a number of ways in addition to success or failure. Many poly people view their relationships as fundamentally based on personal choice, and if the relationship became unhealthy or intolerable, violated boundaries, or no longer met the participants' needs, then the correct response was to modify or end the relationship. Tacit Campo said:

> If you are in a relationship or several relationships then you *choose* to do that, every day, whether you recognize it or not. You can stay because you consciously make that decision or you can just stay because you are on automatic pilot, but that is a choice too.

This consciously engaged choice means that polyamorous people acknowledge their own responsibility for their relationships, with little or no social pressure (from the polyamorous paradigm at least) to either stay together or break up. As a result, poly people ultimately define their relationships as both voluntary and utilitarian, in that they are designed to meet participants' needs. Clearly it is easier to focus on self-responsibility when the people in question are financially self-supporting and do not have children whose lives would be affected by parental separation. Given the framework of those familial and social constraints, poly people attach diverse meanings to the ends or transitional points of relationships.

In my research, three primary definitions of the ends of relationships stood out: success or failure, shifting interests and needs, and change or transition. While each category is distinct, they are not mutually exclusive and often overlap. Fewer of the poly people I interviewed defined their relationship ends in terms of failure, and many more emphasized their shifting needs and interests, and especially the fluid nature of relationships over time.

It Is Really Over: Success and Failure

Some polyamorous relationships last until one of the partners dies, and in that sense they meet the conventional definition of "success" because the family members did not separate from each other during their lives. The Wysses began as a sextet of three couples and evolved significantly over time, losing partners to death and divorce. The original sextet was composed of three legally married couples—Loretta and Albert, Kiyowara and Patrick, and Margret and Tim—who conglomerated into a cohabitational family with older children from previous relationships. After two years of love, fighting, and conciliation, Margret divorced the entire family, including legally divorcing Tim. The resultant group had only just restabilized when Tim was killed in an automobile accident. Even though the surviving spice lost their husband to death, they did not frame it as a "successful" end. Instead of using a success/failure characterization, the Wyss quad emphasized the joy they had with Tim when he was alive, the pain they felt at his death, and how the relative invisibility of their poly widowhood compounded their sense of loss because the monogamous culture at large did not define them as widow/ers.

About the same time Tim was killed in the accident, Kiyowara became pregnant with Albert's child and bore the quad's daughter Kethry. Fourteen very full years later, the Wyss quad became the Wyss triad when Patrick divorced Kiyowara (legally), Albert and Loretta (socially).

Kiyowara characterized the relationship as a success even though it ended:

> I am glad we are coparenting and not married. . . . I certainly can't call it a failure; it was a twenty-year marriage. And I am glad his current choices are not my problem. Any time a relationship ends there is a tendency to view it as a failure. I was very clear that a relationship that had good times and lasted twenty years was not a failure, it just ended. End does not mean fail. That totally invalidates anything good that came out of it. I had a lot of people remind me that it is not a personal failure just because something had run a full cycle and came to its end.

Kiyowara redefined the end of the relationship with Patrick from failure to relief from dealing with his choices and continued contact as coparents. Friends in her poly community "reminded" her that it was not failure but rather the end of a cycle, supporting her redefinition. Such reinforcement allowed these alternate meanings to take on more social gravity and ultimately become solidified as poly social norms that accept the ends of relationships and encourage former lovers to remain friends.

For others, the end of a poly relationship kept the taint of failure in the conventional sense. Although poly community norms encourage people to remain friends with former lovers, some relationships end with such acrimony that former lovers find remaining friends to be neither desirable nor feasible. People whose relationships ended with infuriated distance were more likely to see the end of the relationship as a failure, both in the conventional sense of ending sexual and intimate relations and as a *poly* failure in that they broke community norms dictating continued friendly contact with former lovers as friends.

Jessica, a forty-three-year-old woman and registered nurse, had been in a triad when she was in her mid-thirties with Mira and James, a married couple with two young children. For about a year and a half the triad spent five to seven nights a week together, often at the couple's home engaged in family activities such as making dinner, doing dishes, and bathing and putting the children to bed. When the triad broke up, Jessica reported feeling like they had failed because at the beginning we said that if we were going to be like a family then I would stay connected to the girls, no matter what happened with us [the adults]. And for that time I was definitely, not quite a second mom, but at least an auntie who was around all the time . . . But then when we broke up, I just realized they [Mira and James] were not who I wanted to spend time with and it was awkward to call them or try to talk to the girls. Mira was especially weird on the phone and . . . eventually I just kind of stopped calling, and now it has been years since I have seen them. So I guess in that way it feels like a failure, because we didn't stay connected like we had planned to.

In Jessica's view, the end of the triad was a failure not only because the adults stopped interacting but also because she lost contact with the children she had lovingly cared for over a year and a half.

Because poly relationships can have multiple adults involved, relationships between some members can end while they continue between others. In these cases, some of the people involved may define it as a failure but others may not. Morgan and Clark Majek's family was characteristic of this tendency for some adults to maintain contact even though others stop seeing each other. Morgan and Clark, both white and middle class, met in college and married in their mid-twenties. After several happy years of marriage and the birth of their daughter, they attempted to form a quad with another female/male couple. Six months later it was clear to everyone that the quad was not working, and while they no longer stayed in contact Morgan reported that "I learned a lot from that initial experience so I don't think of it as a failure—it was a learning experience."

Later, when Morgan was pregnant with their second child, she and Clark established another quad with James and Melissa, a couple who had been married for almost ten years. Melissa and James's marriage had been in crisis before, and they had separated for almost six months several years earlier but had reunited prior to meeting Morgan and Clark. James and Morgan fell in love, and Clark and Melissa investigated a relationship but realized, as Clark reported, "we did not have the right chemistry." Melissa was sometimes close to Morgan and Clark and at other times quite distant, but Morgan, Clark, and James established an intimate emotional connection. For five years James, Morgan, Clark, and their two children spent three to six days per week together and shared many family events.

Eventually James and Morgan's relationship soured and, with hurt feelings on both sides, they stopped seeing each other. Clark, however, reported that he and James maintained friendly relations:

> Oh yeah, we get to see him all the time. Either we drive down to [a town about forty-five minutes away] or he comes up here. Actually, usually we go down there, probably every other week or so. I actually get along with James better than Morgan does right now, so it makes sense for me to take [the kids] down to see him. I know the kids miss him a lot so I definitely put effort in to getting them together. I still like him, too, so it is nice for me to see him, though I don't think I would do it nearly as much if it weren't for the kids.

While James and Morgan's relationship fit one definition of failure because they no longer saw each other, the rest of the family maintained a successful relationship with James, if success is defined as remaining in contact. This flexible definition allows for polyaffective relationships in which children can stay in contact with adults who are important to them, even if the adults are no longer in sexually intimate relationships with their parents. In that sense, this expansion of options that allows polys to define the relationships as successful (even though they have "failed") also sustains family connections.

Moving Apart: Diverging Interests and Needs

Some polys like Angela, a thirty-two-year old white woman in the IT industry, emphasized the idea that they were no longer relating to former partners the same way (or possibly at all), but rather:

> moving apart without blame—people change over time and what worked before no longer does, or what was once interesting to everyone is now boring to some of us who are now interested in this new thing. Like [my ex-husband] Mike with his whole anime thing, that holds no interest for me, absolutely none . . . and he has no interest in crafting, which has become really important to me and takes up a lot of my time. There is no judgment or shame for changing from the people we were when we met at SCA[12] all those years ago, we are just not who we used to be and don't fit together as well anymore.

Like Angela, people in this category emphasized divergent interests and decreasing time spent with partners who had formerly shared more interests as the key factors that influenced how they defined their shifting relationships. Poly people often have full lives and hectic schedules, so time is at a premium, and how people "spend" it frequently indicates their relational allegiances. If partners spend a lot of time doing different things, then they may develop divergent social lives, resulting in less overlap in social circles and decreasing importance for some relationships as others increase in intimacy and time together. This shift is not necessarily failure; for some it is simply change.

Some poly people discussed the shifting definitions of relationships as they ended or changed once they were no longer meeting participants' needs. If communication and renegotiation did not address the lack, and the relationship remained unsatisfying or defective despite attempts to address the problems, then poly people either reconfigured their expectations or ended the relationship in that form. Jared, a forty-six-year-old divorced father of two and a health care professional, linked his recent breakup with a girlfriend to the fact that the relationship was no longer meeting needs for either of them.

> When I first started dating Janice we were pretty much on the same page with our needs. She has a primary who is out of town a lot and wanted a close secondary, and I am not ready for a primary but wanted a close secondary, so it was great that way for a while. Then she started dating Erika and Mark and began spending more and more time with them to the point that I only got to see her, from two or three nights a week sometimes down to every other week or something. That just wasn't enough for me—I didn't need to move in with her or anything, but twice a month? I mean, come on. So when it became clear that she needed more freedom and I needed more intimacy, we split.

Characteristic of the many poly people who identified the ability for multiple relationships to meet a variety of needs as one of the primary reasons they became polyamorous, Jared and Janice had begun dating to meet their needs for companionship and sex. When the amount or kind of companionship—or any other basic motivator for the specific relationship—no longer met their needs, people like Jared reported "moving on to other relationships that will meet my needs better, at least I hope." Polys in this category often saw the relationship as ending or at least changing dramatically to something far less than it had been previously. Even so, it was not a failure as conventionally defined—rather acceptance that people change and no one need be at fault.

Not Really the End: Changes and Continuity

For some polys, simply no longer having sex did not signal the end of a relationship, but rather a shift to a new phase. In these cases, the emphasis of the relationship changed to a nonsexual interaction, but the emotional and social connections remained continuous. JP Amore—a sixty-eight-year old woman with five children, eight grandchildren, and one great-grandchild—had been married eight times, four of them to her first husband, Richard, with whom she retained an emotionally intimate, nonsexual relationship. Reflecting on her long and varied relationship with Richard, which began in high school when they "got pregnant and got married immediately—both of us were virgins and we got pregnant on our first time, imagine that!" JP reported that

> we have a tremendous closeness. We've always been able to talk. Intellectual connection, spiritual connection. Just a very intimate relationship. We've got all of this history together, grandkids, a great-grandchild even! I went to Houston not too long ago, and we celebrated the fiftieth anniversary of our wedding. We got to celebrate all of it!

While JP harbored no illusions that Richard was perfect, stating that he has a "multifaceted personality, a wonderful person on one hand, and a male chauvinist controlling jerk on the other," she was able to preserve the positive aspects of the relationship and celebrate a fiftieth wedding anniversary with her long-time companion, even though they had both been married to other people over the years. Their relationship overflowed the boundaries of conventional marriage, and their emotional continuity overshadowed the fact that they no longer had sex.

True to form in poly communities who shape language to reflect their relationships,[13] some polys reject or redefine the concept of the "ex." Laszlo, a man in his mid-thirties, commented that the notion of *ex* is ill-defined unless you have a social context, like (serial) monogamy where at least some "privileged" relationship statuses are single-person-only exclusive. That is, if you don't *have* to "break up" to be with someone else, then attempting to categorize *all* of the people from your past relationships as "ex-pickrelationshiplabel" is kinda goofy/nonsensical . . . I can see using the "ex" label structure for relationships that were abusive and continued contact would be unhealthy, but if instead they're still-or-once-again a friend, why focus on what they aren't anymore instead of what they are right now?

While Gabrielle, a woman in her mid-forties, was clear that "I am not best buddies with all of my exes, not by any stretch," she nonetheless asserted that

> I have other former lovers that I suppose ex would be *a* term for. But, I don't think of them as exes. We were lovers and now we're friends, and ex just seems kind of a weird way to think of someone I'm close to and care about. The real difference here, I think, is that the changes in relationship tended to have a much more gentle evolution rather than "official" breakups.

Rather than an "official breakup," the relationship went through a transition and entered a new phase. Emphasizing the present and continuing existence of the relationship, Gabrielle and Laszlo had room to define former lovers as friends with whom they remained close and caring.

As in most relationship styles, this varies by relationship and depends on how people handle transitions. Sorcia, a Native American woman in her mid-thirties, commented:

> Of course, it depends on the person. Of my former triad—one parent is . . . not even on the remotest of friendly terms with the other two of us. On the other hand, my ex-wife and I are still good friends. We do the holidays together with the kids, get together regularly for dinner and generally weather our ups and downs. We consider each other to be family. She moved in with a boyfriend last fall and one of her pre-reqs was being OK with our familial connection. It's turned out much better than I ever expected and it's pretty cool.

People in poly relationships create a range of relationship outcomes and a wide array of meanings from which to select. Some follow a conventional pattern of alienation when a sexual relationship ends, while others forge views that define former partners as continued intimates, or "chosen kin."[14]

Shifting the crux of the relationship from sexuality to emotional intimacy can foster more connected and cooperative coparenting because it allows for continued and cooperative relationships among adults. While Michael, a father in his mid-fifties, and his coparent divorced fifteen years ago, they continued to cohabit for six years afterward, and

> we have stayed in frequent contact, taking vacations together (sometimes with our other lovers), continuing to raise our kids in close concert, and recently undertook a major multiyear project together (though we were on opposite coasts). She recently told me that she was thinking about her best friends in the whole world, and of the four people she identified, one was me and another was my long-term nesting partner.

Michael reported that his nonsexual relationships had been crucial to his life and well-being, and that being in poly relationships allowed him the unique opportunity to not only remain emotionally intimate in a cooperative, coparenting relationship but also "being free *not* to have sex with your intimate partner(s)."

> I have these amazing relationships that were once sexual, and in the monogamous world, if I stayed as close as I am with these women, it would be likely to cause substantial stress, or at least some negative social pressure. And each of my emotionally intimate relationships can be sexual or not, sometimes shifting one way or another, without damaging our basic relationship. In a monogamous world, if I stopped being sexual with my primary partner, this would either be a major source of distress, or might end the relationship entirely. As a poly person, I don't feel uniquely responsible to meet my partner's sexual needs. If it best serves our intimacy not to be sexual, either temporarily or permanently, then we can do that without any other *necessary* consequences.

Michael emphasized the changing nature of relationships over time, as sexual interest waxed and waned due to the vigor of youth, having children, shifting circumstances, and passage along the life course.

> Over the years, I've had two lovers, both previously *very* sexually assertive, who found that menopause made sex less interesting and less enjoyable for them. They suspect that this may change back at some point, when their hormones settle down, but in the meantime, sex is pretty much off the table for them with all their lovers. This didn't change our connection at all, though. We still sleep (sleep!) together from time to time, do naked cuddling, and have intense, intimate conversations. We just don't have sex, as it is usually conceived of.

Regardless of whether this relationship phase was truly the end of their sexual connection or simply a hiatus, Michael's long-term relationships with his partners continued despite changing sexual and relational circumstances.

7

BENEFITS OF POLYAMOROUS FAMILY LIFE

People in polyamorous families identified a variety of benefits that accompanied their family style. These included honesty and emotional intimacy among family members and a number of benefits associated with increased resources that come with multiple-adult families, such as more money, accommodating disabilities, personal time for parents, more attention for children, and abundant role models for children. Some children identified their parents' ability to remain friendly as advantageous, and many polys discussed the advantages of an expanded chosen family.

HONESTY AND EMOTIONAL INTIMACY AMONG FAMILY MEMBERS

Parents emphasized honesty with their children as a key element of their overall relationship philosophy and parenting strategy. Poly parents routinely use honesty in a variety of discussions, ranging from their own shortcomings or mistakes to age-appropriate answers to questions about sexuality. Polyamorous parents often characterize honesty as the primary factor that cultivates emotional intimacy because, as Brad (a white father of two) commented, "the kids get to see us as real people too." He continued:

We [Brad's wife and their boyfriend] make mistakes, and we cop to them. We tell them what is really happening in our lives, and they do the same with us. Of course there is a line—we don't tell them anything about our sex lives or adult relationship details, but we tell them the most truth we can and still remain in the parental role.

Evelyn and Mark Coach, both white, middle-class professionals, were in a polyamorous marriage for eighteen years and similarly focused on being truthful with Martine, their older daughter from Mark's previous marriage, and Annabelle, the daughter of their union. Mark asserted:

We're just very straight with the kids and I just don't know any other way to be. Whatever Martine asks I always answer it completely straight. Annabelle, too, but just in a different way. Something that is easier for her to understand, whereas I give Martine the longer version.

Similarly, Alexander, a white machinist/mechanic and father of two, emphasized honesty. He and his wife, Yansa, an African American health care provider, told their adolescent daughter, Chantal (from Alexander's previous marriage), the truth about everything, including sex. Alexander detailed Chantal's reaction to seeing a movie scene with women kissing:

My daughter goes, "Ooooo, that's disgusting!" And . . . Yansa says, "How can that be disgusting? Every woman you know is like that." And you could see the gears grinding in her head and finally one of them engages and she goes, "But you mean, you are?" And Yansa's like, "Yes." And then Chantal stopped for a little while and another gear engaged and it was like, "You mean my mother?" Yansa goes, "Yes." And then she decided uh, yeah, it's not all that bad.

Such candor about sexuality contributes to a sex-positive environment where children feel comfortable asking questions that might seem taboo in other settings. Some parents reported that they, and their children, became sources of sex education for entire peer groups of adolescents. Kay, a white woman with five children who identified as bisexual/queer/pan-sexual, commented that my older kids' friends come to us a lot for, you know, since they know we have this open relationship and we're poly and I'm bisexual. I've had a lot of their friends ask me about their relationships or how to come out, or handle multiple relationships, or how to even manage some of their friendship relationships when everyone isn't getting along. Also about birth control and things like that, things that they feel like they can't talk to their own parents about.

Kay celebrated her ability to offer candid, sex-positive advice because "these kids see me as a relationship expert." True to polyamorous form, Kay used honesty as one of her most valued relationship tools in order to foster emotional intimacy with her own children and their friends.

Even when parents are not immediately honest with their children, if they are honest later it can still contribute to emotional intimacy. Mandy, a white college student and worker in the hospitality industry, said that her parents had been in a polyamorous relationship when she was growing up in a small town in the Midwest. They never discussed it with her, but Mandy reported that she

knew something was going on. And I was always like OK, Mom, I know you are hiding something from me. Just come out with it. And it took them a while but once I went away to college she told me the truth and now we are a lot closer. Almost like more of a friend relationship, a lot more emotionally intimate than we used to be. And we are a lot closer than she is with my sister, who just couldn't handle it. I mean, she lives in a small town and trains horses, and I moved to this big city to go to college and I work in the city. I am just more open-minded than she is. And my mom knew she could tell me the truth, and I'm glad she did because now we are a lot closer now that there are no more secrets.

Marcus Amore linked honesty and choice to significant personal advantages associated with poly families.

One of the main advantages is knowing you have choices. Understanding that I have a choice and that I do not have to conform to society, being able to decide for myself. . . . The freedom of choice is in many ways the definition of being human in my opinion. So because I've always been presented with the freedom of choice rather than anything about trying to follow a societal norm—and this was open to me because of [my parents'] honesty—I feel that I have had the freedom and as such, all those choices led to a positive life for me.

Throughout his interview, Marcus elaborated on his reasons for feeling lucky to have grown up in a polyamorous family, such as a relaxed atmosphere without the tension of trying to hide anything, the freedom to think anything without any topics being off limits, and his ability to "make some very good friends, and very true friends who do not abandon me just because I'm different or anything like that." Most importantly, he expressed a deep conviction that freedom, honesty, and choice pervade the true human condition, and he felt that being in a polyamorous family allowed him unique access to this compelling humanity:

> In my opinion, this is what sets humans apart from many other species on the planet. Not our advanced technology, not our "superiority" over them. Frankly, it's our freedom. Unfortunately, I feel that it's also a major lack of that. Not so much in appearance as it is in mentality. That is causing a lot of our problems. The people who have done the most for the world have been very free thinkers. So, I believe that the freedom of choice, the freedom of thought are the best things about being human. Unfortunately, I feel that that's absent in a lot of people who simply try to conform to society. So I feel like that's the advantage. That's what I enjoy about my family.

Similarly, Kethry Wyss thought that she was closer to her parents because of their acceptance of and engagement with her—something she saw in sharp contrast with her peers' parents.

> My parents are aware of my life. We have a good dialog, there is nothing I would keep from them. We are just very open people; there is no need to hide anything. There is nothing I could do that would cause my parents to freak out and ground me. They might be worried about me, but they would not freak and send me to a mental institution like one of my friends' parents did. They did not understand what she was doing so they sent her to an institution in Nevada and did not tell her. Some of my friends, things are bad for them at home, they can't and don't want to talk to their parents. It is kinda

sad; they don't think they can trust their parents. In a lot of cases they are right to not trust their parents, that they can't tell their parents things is legitimate, they should not tell their parents stuff. I can tell my parents things, there is really nothing I should hide from my parents.

In this case, Kethry thought that her poly family was far more advantageous to her than a conventional monogamous family would be because it encouraged parents and children to be honest with each other. In that same interview Kethry elaborated on her parents' involvement and investment in her life:

My friends all want my parents to be their parents because my parents are cool, they go to concerts and stuff, they take me cool places and do cool things with me. I am always taken aback when my friends say they have never even been to a concert, and I have been going since I was a wee one. Lots of steampunk, goth, industrial. My mom (Loretta) took me to *The Rocky Horror Picture Show*, for goodness sake. I have the rockstar parents! My friends are Facebook friends with my parents. My parents don't control what I say on Facebook, and my mom posted a picture of us going to *Rocky Horror*—it was fun. . . . [Good parenting] is being willing to listen to your children, to really listen, and to not shun them for being interested in something. I got into anime, and my mama (Kiyowara) has helped me sew costumes and takes me thrift shopping for costume pieces. My other friends' mom just does not understand it and it keeps my friend from being as involved. My mama also helps me dye my hair—pink, red, blue, black, maybe purple next. She also helped my friend dye his hair green cause his mom wouldn't. She was OK with him dying his hair but had never dyed hair before so mom helped him dye his hair green.

Kethry and Marcus both saw their family lives and relationships with their parents as fostering positive, authentic connections. Polyamory, with its emphasis on communication and honesty, helps children in poly families to feel connected to their parents in a way Kethry and Marcus did not see among their peers in monogamous families. In that way, poly families are especially advantageous for children who value emotional intimacy with their parents. Adults and children in poly families as a whole are optimistic about their familial styles and the impact multiple-partner relating has on their lives, prizing especially what they saw as tremendous emotional intimacy with family members.

SHARED RESOURCES

Poly parents routinely mention the ability of multiple partners to meet a variety of familial needs as one of the most important benefits to poly-amorous family life. From shared income to increased personal time for adults and more attention for children, having numerous adults in the family allows members to distribute tasks so that (ideally) no one person has to take the brunt of family care.

Money

Pooling financial resources frequently results in more money for every-one. Larger family units are often able to keep a parent at home be-cause they have multiple adults doing waged work. The Wyss quad, for example, was able to afford a stay-at-home parent for their daughter Kethry's entire childhood, even in the notoriously expensive California Bay Area. As a computer programmer with a stable income, Albert was the family's primary economic support. Cycling through self-employ-ment, professional managerial positions, and college attendance, each of the other three adults took primary parenting responsibility at differ-ent times, and they shared parenting and transit duties once Kethry was in high school. The assurance of a predictable income granted the quad the flexibility of rotating the position of full-time parenthood, enabling other adults to be selective when looking for work, in establishing busi-nesses, and in pursuing higher education.

The Wysses, however, also experienced the negative side of shared income when two of their three workers lost jobs in an economic down-turn, leaving Albert the sole wage earner. Albert reported that "it felt like a lot of pressure . . . everyone was counting on me and it made me really nervous. What if I lost my job too?" Other single-wage-earner families face similar fears, but fewer have the flexibility of multiple reserve wage earners to get jobs and simultaneously retain a full-time parent. While these larger groupings require a lot of food, large houses, and multiple cars, their pooled resources grant greater flexibility and save money on expenses such as child care and separate dwellings.

Social Stimulation (and Loot)

Children in these families also see the family's pooled resources as an advantage. Zane Lupine reminisced about the glee of having such a large extended family when it was time to receive gifts as a child. "When I was young I guess more presents at Christmas. More people. Just more people in general. I liked it as a little kid, cause I liked having people around. And great loot for birthdays and Christmas, with three parents and so many grandparents."

Adam, Jonathan, and Zoe Hadaway agreed that the increased resources were great for the children in the family, and to the parents as well.

> Jonathan: They're probably not as bored as they used to be. They have a lot more people to actually talk with.

> Elisabeth: Who used to be bored?

> Adam: Our parents. One of them would be at work and the other would be at home with four-plus kids. It just became aggravating sometimes. It's a little better for all of them to just be there for each other, I think . . . and we are all more open-minded, too.

> Zoe: Yeah, technically we are an alternative family. Having that on our side, we're not against the alternative lifestyle. Which makes, in my opinion, if you're open to other kinds of life, that's going to open so many doors to you. That's going to make so many more opportunities for friendships. Through friendships you get contacts and through contacts you get financial opportunities that you may not be able to pass up. That's my mind-set.

Overall, poly family members said sharing resources was the single most important advantage to their family style. In addition to the more general financial and personal resources, they identified other advantages such as accommodating family members with disabilities and allowing parents to have more personal time for themselves.

Accommodating Disabilities

Several respondents mentioned how useful it was to have multiple partners when dealing with disabilities, either their own or their children's.
Heidi Ballard reported that she occasionally had "anxiety severe enough
that it made going places uncomfortable, and sometimes even staying
home alone can be uncomfortable." While she did not require "someone constantly holding my hand, I don't need a babysitter," Heidi did
experience significant angst dealing with her occasionally debilitating
anxiety. She explained how her polyamorous relationship had improved
her life and made it easier to manage her periods of extreme anxiety:

> And then when Jason moved in it came as such a relief. 'Cause he
> works at home a lot of the time, and just having someone there
> during the day when I was home with the kids, I could hear him in
> the other room or just chat for a few minutes, it brought my anxiety
> level down quite a bit. And if I'm not up for going out but don't want
> to be alone at home, we can still do things or get groceries or whatev-
> er because there's someone to be home with me and someone to go
> do whatever needs to be done. It just works out better that way.
> George has more freedom to come and go or stay late at work or do
> something on the way home because Jason is here, I'm not alone
> with the kids in the house.

With the accommodations her polyamorous family was able to provide, Heidi's anxiety felt much more manageable for the entire family.
George reported that he "just feel[s] better knowing Jason is here with
Heidi and the kids, that she's more comfortable, I don't feel so pressed
to rush home." Jason was similarly enthusiastic about the arrangement,
saying, "I like spending time with Heidi, so it works great for me too."
    Dillon, son of the Kenmore quad, had what his mother, Natalie,
termed a "cognitive processing disorder" that resulted in speech delays
and interaction issues like avoidance of eye contact. His disability wasn't
clearly diagnosed yet because Dillon was only six years old at the time
of the interview and had not yet had some of the learning or cognitive
tests the Kenmores planned to schedule for the future. A quiet and
gentle child, Dillon played with action figures while I sat on the floor
next to him and asked him questions.

Elisabeth: So what do you think of living with Iris and William too [in addition to parents Dax and Natalie]?

Dillon: Good.

Elisabeth: What's good about it?

Dillon: There's always someone here [pause] just in case.

Elisabeth: In case of what?

Dillon: If I run in the street or, or, or can't find my way home, or [pause] they will always come get me.

Elisabeth: Has that happened, do you ever run away accidentally?

Dillon: No.

Elisabeth: But if it did, they would come find you?

Dillon: Yeah, they will always come.

When he said this, Dillon radiated calm and smiled up at his father, Dax, sitting in a chair to his left. While he had some difficulty formulating the words to describe how his behavior might be unpredictable even to himself, it was abundantly clear to me that the four adults' combined attention provided Dillon with a safety net that made his amorphous disability less frightening and more manageable for him and for the adults in his life.

Personal Time

It is clear that, in general, polyamorists perceive themselves to be happier when they are getting more of their needs met,[1] and they are able to get a wider range of needs met through multiple partners. This same dynamic appears to extend to nonsexual familial relationships as well. When the Wyss quad had Kethry, their ability to distribute parenting meant that Patrick Wyss could parent full time and "retain my sanity." After spending all day with a rambunctious toddler who "did better when she stayed home, [because she had] major fits in public for a little while," Patrick felt harried and claustrophobic. Patrick reported that when Kiyowara or Albert arrived home one or both would "take over with Kethry and I would split, go ride my bike in the foothills for an hour or two . . . It saved me, I never could have done it without it." The ability to leave Kethry with others allowed Patrick to meet his need for time away from a demanding toddler. For the Wyss quad, this made a very challenging period in the parenting cycle much easier than it would have been with only two (or fewer) parents.

The Tree triad, composed of Bjorn, Gene, and Leah—all professionals or academicians in their mid-thirties—similarly found multiple parents to be invaluable when caring for their infant son, Will. Leah said that everyone got more sleep because there were more people to take night shifts:

> As far as having Will goes, it has made a huge difference to have multiple parents, and multiple grandparents. Gene and Bjorn took turns staying at the hospital or going home for a full night's sleep just after Will was born, and being able to be well rested has made a world of difference not only then but Will's whole life so far. The difference has not been quite as big for me because I was there at the hospital full time after I had Will, but overall spreading out the parenting has been great. Despite only getting four or five hours of sleep for five days or so right when we had Will, we were all really calm and excited about meeting this new little person. We were lucky enough to have a hospital room all to ourselves so we ended up with an extra bed in the room so daddy or papa could get a real sleep while they were at the hospital with us [Leah and Will], which helped a lot.

Bjorn agreed with Leah, putting the poly parenting experience in context with some of his other friends who had children around the same time:

> It has been amusing having monogamous friends who first asked questions about polyamory, like "isn't that complicated or a lot of work?" Then as we all got to child-rearing age our friends have changed their tune or seemed a little jealous and talk about how wonderful it would be to have more parents—single parents want more help and the couples want another parent as well. It's a full-

time job for the three of us; we can't even imagine doing it with fewer adults. Our friends tease us but wish they had more help too.

In addition to more time to themselves and spreading parenting around, Gene said that having a baby in a polyamorous situation seemed to help him get dates with other women.

> Before we got pregnant I was only in one other relationship that ended and I chose not to look for another knowing that I wanted to devote all my energy and flexibility to that [having a baby]. Once I determined what life with a kid was like and got things more under control (or as much control as things ever are once you have a kid), I went back to dating again. It's going great, the people that I have been dating have been really interested in hearing about and meeting Will. No complications. If anything, it is something that people find interesting—the kind of people I would be interested in dating see it as a bonus, intrinsically appealing and interesting—"How do you do that?" So it has led a couple of people to contact me. Women are reaching out to me on my online dating profile and they have reached out to me seeing Will as something interesting.

Not only was the new father still fully engaged in life in a way he saw his monogamous counterparts trying and mostly failing to achieve but also being in a polyamorous family actually made Gene more appealing to women who then wanted to date him.

Attention for Children

Another important advantage poly people mention is the considerable attention available to children when families with multiple adults pool their resources. Many parents say that their children's lives, experiences, and self-concepts are richer for the multiple loving adults in their families. Joya Starr said polyamory was beneficial for her son Gideon because

> there's more attention for the kids . . . It takes five adults to raise a kid and one of those adults is just around to take care of mom. And let me tell you, a happy mom is a good mom. If mom gets enough sleep then everyone is in much better shape.

Having multiple adults in the household benefitted both children and adults, Joya observed, because happy and well-rested parents provided better care for children. Not only did children get more attention from a wider variety of adults, but adults who were able to support each other (ideally) parented more effectively.

Some respondents connected this increased attention with a feeling of community. Emmanuella Ruiz identified the connection to chosen family her poly family provided as crucial to her children's well-being:

> It gives my children a sense of community. They've not had reliable grandparents. They don't have cousins or the typical biological extended family. But they have a big, happy, productive, healthy family nonetheless, and it is a chosen family. They know each person's relationship to them the same way they would know if they were first or second cousins, aunts or uncles . . . The sense of extended community is the most important thing in respect to my children.

Emmanuella saw her children as gaining both a community in lieu of their unreliable grandparents and a sense of how to construct chosen relationships that contributed to a healthy sense of intimacy.

In addition to a sense of extended community contributing to children's well-being, some polys feel that their assistance to poly parents provided what one woman at a party jokingly referred to as "fresh horses," referring to the Pony Express message service operating from 1860 to 1861 in the Western United States that provided riders with a new mount every ten miles to get the messages to their destinations more rapidly.[2] Kristine saw herself as relief for Mark and Evelyn Coach in the demanding task of parenting their (then) elementary-aged daughter, Annabelle:

> Of course, I had it easier, in a way. It was easier to make her a priority when I was there, not being a full-time parent, because she really is a handful. The time I had with her could be just with her, focusing on being with her and not trying to do other things at the same time.

This allowed for Evelyn and Mark to do paid work, complete household tasks like making dinner or cleaning, and have a few rare moments of personal time. It also provided Annabelle with the undivided attention of an adoring adult who was not harried by thoughts of needing to do something else. Sharing child care tasks and parental resources proved beneficial in a variety of ways to both children and adults in poly families.

Role Models for Children

One of the major advantages poly parents mention is the plentiful positive role modeling available to children in poly families. These role models include ethical considerations like honesty, a willingness to meet other's needs, and careful communication and negotiation. Perhaps most importantly, parents emphasize the relationships between their children, partners, and friends as sources of personal role modeling through life examples and advice. Melody Lupine lived for seven years in a triad with two men: Cristof, her husband of eighteen years, and Quentin, the couple's long-time friend-turned-lover whom Melody considered her husband. Melody noted that Quentin functioned as a positive example for her son, Pete (the biological child of Melody and Cristof):

> Quentin is another male role model in Pete's life. He has his dad and that's his dad, but here is another man in his life or other men in his life and this is what they do and their acceptance of him. And so which I think is very beneficial for a young man to have those different role models and know that, Pete knows that he could go to them at any time for anything if he needed something, he knew that they were available.

The availability of multiple adults not only provided a broad range of role models but it also gave children in poly families access to nonparental trusted adults with whom to discuss things the children might not wish to tell their parents.

Zoe Hadaway similarly saw multiple adults as a positive source of attention and role models:

> I think having four parents is the best thing about being in a poly family. You know, some people at school are like "I hate that my parents are divorced and I hate that I have all these extra parents now!" and I'm like, well, minus the divorce part, I can't say that having more parents is all that bad. I always feel like if Gwenyth, my

biological mother, is busy then I can go to Tammy or I can go to Phil. Or to my dad. I don't just have two options now; I have four. It sort of makes trying to find advice a little bit easier. You know that each parent has their own specific forte of advice. Like Phil's mechanical. Dad's business. Mom's in the house, as is Tammy. Tammy's more artsy and technology. Mom's very clean oriented, organization. It's nice, you get lots of different things from the different parents.

For Zoe, growing up in a polyamorous family provided a wealth of role models and advice from the expanded number of parents.

Similarly, Cole Cypress explained how more numerous authority figures provided him with a greater diversity of parental options, avenues for support, and a profusion of role models. Cole said that he was a "wild thing" when he was in sixth and seventh grade, and while his parents would "scream bloody murder at me," he appreciated how his parent's girlfriend Bettina "had a different way of going about her business with me. She would react very calmly and know exactly what to do and the exact right punishment. And it would still be really hard for me, but it helped me learn my lesson better. And it felt more fair." Cole elaborated on an incident in which he got in trouble at school and Bettina created a creative punishment for him:

> There was one incident where I took, well, part of it was an accident and part of it kind of wasn't. I accidentally forgot two pocket knives in my backpack. But the fact that didn't make it an accident was that I started kinda showing them off, but then I got caught with them, and I got punished for it. At school they took the knives away and gave me a very strict warning, which was pretty traditional at the private school. And my parents heard about it and they of course were very upset. But Bettina of course had a different way of punishing me . . . she made me build a dog house using only the pocket knives. And after about three days of that she made me stop because I was injuring my hands because the knives kept slipping. But I never used a pocket knife after that. And of course my parents wanted to ground me for a month and take away all of my privileges and stuff like that. But Bettina would always step in and calm them down and say this stuff really politely and quietly.

Cole felt that he had benefitted from Bettina's alternate way of handling both family conflict and discipline, as well as gaining greater social interaction and diversity of role models.

PARENTS' ABILITY TO REMAIN FRIENDLY

Some children whose families have experienced divorce but stayed in social contact said they valued their parents' ability to remain friends, even after a divorce. Speaking of her parents' divorce, Kethry Wyss expressed mixed feelings but ultimately felt that the divorce had not changed things much for her at all:

> It was a bit of a change now that there are two houses instead of one, but not really that big of a deal. The first thing I said when they told me they were getting divorced was, "now the shouting will stop." It got better immediately after they decided to divorce. By the time everything was through the court system they were back to being friends, Mama (Kiyowara) and Poppa (Patrick) were friends again. . . . In terms of being a kid of a divorce, I was dealt a really good deal in terms of being with Mama and Poppa—even when they were fighting they weren't out of control. They would take a deep breath and even walk away for a bit if they needed to cool down. They were really rational about their fights, as rational as you can be in that situation. Dealing with the courts and everything they became friends again and they can still hang out in the same room. Watching as Lucia (Patrick's new wife) has struggled with her ex-husband, about their son Evan and that whole debacle, as well as some of Nina and Paton's issues with their kids and their ex-spouses—I was dealt a very very good hand with parents who were able to become friends again afterwards. They are still friends. The other divorces, just, some, like, these kids I know with their stepmother and their dad, their stepmother is not a very nice person. . . . it was hard to watch from the sidelines to see how the daughters and the mom were taking it.

While children in other families who divorce may experience cooperative parenting after a divorce, Kethry saw her peers and their parents struggling far more than her parents did. She reported that she was able to see Patrick regularly, even though he had moved out of the quad's house:

> Usually, like last year [I saw my dad] four times a week or so, he would pick me up from school on Tuesdays and Fridays and then I would ride the train home on Thursday and he would pick me up and take me to the game, bring me back afterwards. We would play Dungeons and Dragons role-play for like three hours, 7 to 10. We still play, we both have characters and we have been gaming with a group of people for the last three years. We have also gone to a gaming convention together, and I game with my friends as well . . . On Saturdays Daddy and Poppa and I go to Costco and come back and watch *Doctor Who* or *Torchwood*. I see Poppa several days every week. I hang out with him and watch TV at his house . . . Special things we do regularly together. He and Mama are friends with Mommy and Daddy too, so it is not like it is awkward visitation or anything.

The fact that Kethry was routinely able to see Patrick several days a week was clearly advantageous to her—she spoke with relish of the time she spent with him—and to Patrick himself, because he made a significant amount of time to spend with his daughter every week. This ability to retain positive relationships is advantageous for parents who wish to stay connected with their children after divorce, as well.

BUILDING CHOSEN KINSHIP NETWORKS

Fundamental to poly families, the option to build relationships outside of conventional frameworks is a hallmark of polyamory. While the sexual relationships polys establish with each other get the most attention from the media—in part because they distinguish polyamory from monogamy and friendship, and in part because they are the most sensational aspect of the family—they are not the only or even most important aspect of poly relationships. Respondents note that the emotional or affective elements of their relationships are what make poly families really work or not. Much like heterosexual families, poly families spend far more time hanging out together, doing homework, making dinner, carpooling, folding laundry, and having family meetings or relationship talks than they do having sex. Sexuality is not the heart of the family: without positive emotional relationships, a sexual relationship alone is often insufficient to sustain a complex, long-term relationship. Polyaffectivity, or the nonsexual emotional ties that bind people in poly families together, is far more important to the overall family connection than is any sexual connection between or among adults.

Children's Active Construction of Kinship Networks

Some children told me they actively constructed their own chosen family networks, either by establishing friendships with people they met through their parents or going beyond their parent's social networks and establishing connections with people they felt like they could trust. In some cases children from different families would meet each other at various poly events (the summer campout was a popular meeting spot for kids) and form lasting bonds, and in other cases their connections would be with others outside of the poly community. Zina Campo said that she found her mother Lexi's polyamorous relationships to be advantageous on a number of levels, one of the most important is discussed in the following:

> Zina: It has actually brought me one of my closer friends, too, so, because of the social networking my mother does and has relationships with other people, one of the people who she's friends with is actually my friend's mom, so, it's really cool. Most of the people she's in relationships with are just kind of too cool, I like being around them. One of them even introduced me to someone I think is totally awesome, even though she's in her thirties now, we have become really good friends. . . . I met her because she was a partner of one of my mom's partners and she and my mom were possibly going to be partners at some point or something, but, I don't know. But she's really awesome, it's really cool. When my mom says that she's visiting I get really excited and jump up and down like yay, I get to see her!

> Elisabeth: So what do you two do together, how do you connect?

> Zina: Go shopping, go get coffee or something, or walk our dogs together. Pretty much anything that we can. Friend stuff. . . . Mom has brought another one of her partners home besides Blake, and

one of his partners, and the awesome friend who is one of her partners and one of my friends now, and she brought home one of her
friends who is just a friend, and probably more that I can't remember
right now. She brings home people occasionally, kind of spread out,
so it is kind of a special occasion. I like it when she brings people
home with her, living out in the middle of nowhere it's kind of cool
when anyone comes over at all, so um it's also really cool that I get to
meet people that she is interested in or friends with or maybe partners or whatever, and I get to see them through, I tell her if I
approve or not. It may not change what she does about it, it's usually
in a positive way 'cause I usually approve of them.

Zina Campo not only established enduring friendships with people
she met in her polyamorous community but she also took an active role
in creating her own family by screening her mother's partners and telling her mother "if I approve or not." In so doing, she experienced
significant personal and emotional advantages to being in a poly family,
and she came to conceive of and possibly even exert a degree of control
over the construction of her family that children in many conventional
families would not even consider. These findings confirm Riggs's conclusions that children in sexual minority families, and especially polyamorous or same-sex families, often act as agents who intentionally co-
create their families in unconventional ways.[3]

Family Expansion

For these families, an important part of creating new forms of family is
investing themselves in relationships outside of the biological or legal
connections usually used to determine family status—what scholars
have called *chosen kin* or *chosen family*.[4] An only child, Cole Cypress
felt that being in a poly family had provided him with a wider range of
family relationships with his parents' partner Bettina's children, who
took on sibling roles with Cole in his family. Cole said that

I learned a lot from the kids, too. Because I've always been an only
child, I've always wanted a brother. It was always an older brother.
Or a younger sister. But I ended up getting two older sisters and an
older brother. And I actually, at some points I was really close with
the brother, Caz, Bettina's son . . . whenever my teachers asked me

why I would swear so much I would always always blame Caz. I would always blame him because he would swear tons. He went to a public school. He was raised in a society where, Bettina raised him to swear smart but still he sweared a lot. And he would always act out and be a smart alec. I always acted a lot like him, I always looked to him as an older brother. At some points he was my idol, you know. The only difference is that, by seventh grade, he was the cool kid that could get away with anything. He was still doing well in school and I was the uncool kid that was swearing and getting in trouble and not going anywhere . . . He was always a huge football player, that's a big reason of why he got out of stuff was because he was athletic and I wasn't. He was a huge linebacker, defensive end or whatever he's doing right now. And I always looked up to that and he always loved playing football. He was always really athletic; he was always at the gym. He was the first to take me to the gym, and showed me the ropes. And now he's, I think he got a full scholarship down at [Prestigious University], uh, on a football scholarship, even though he's pretty smart.

From a big brother useful as a role model and a pal to "show him the ropes" to a handy scapegoat for taking the blame for misbehavior, Cole forged a brotherly relationship with Bettina's son, Caz. Cole saw this unusual opportunity for an only child to establish siblingesque relationships as an advantage associated with his parent's polyamorous relationships.

Otherfathering

While the father has been considered the most important or "real" parent in some periods of history,[5] contemporary society in the United States is firmly in the mother's camp when it comes to assigning primary parenting roles. The fact that child care remains a "working mother's issue" speaks volumes about the amount of responsibility society expects fathers—working or not—to take for their children's daily maintenance. Even in multiple-partner families, it is generally the multiple wives who help care for each other's children, and the children caring for each other, as opposed to numerous adult men present in the family to care for the children. Scholars use the term *othermothering*[6] to describe the care work women do for children with whom they share no biological or legal connection. Although Collins used the term in reference to women of African descent or with an Afrocentric world-view caring for each other's children directly by providing meals and clothing or indirectly through offering advice or support,[7] othermothering has some flexibility to be used for men who take on the same role, but it is not generally applied to men.

I argue that polyamory provides men with a unique opportunity to form lasting relationships with children who are not their biological progeny—to become *otherfathers*. Very few of the polyamorous otherfathers are of African descent, so the term does not have racial parity with Collins's use of othermothers,[8] but the emotional and caretaking intent is similar in that each cares for children who are not their own. For instance, Warren Bien considers himself a father of three girls, though only two of them are biologically and legally related to him. He and his ex-wife, Julie, had two daughters—Rebecca and Callie—during their polyamorous marriage, and Julie had another daughter (Macy) with her then-boyfriend, now-husband Andrew during that same time. While Macy is not Warren's biological child, she is his daughters' sister through their mother and, as Warren put it, "a child of my heart. I love her like she is my own, and she calls me her papa bear." Warren said that "my partner Estella and her legal husband Devon are thinking about having kids, and they have asked me what role I would expect to play if they do. I would see myself as a coparent, at least as active as I am in Macy's life. I wouldn't have any legal or genetic tie to any of their kids, but I would still want to be their papa bear."

Similarly, James Majek reported that he had "come as close as I will ever get" to fatherhood through his association with his then-girlfriend Morgan's children, Heather and Brady:

> I am hard-pressed to come up with a negative. I love those kids and they love me. I will never forget being out camping with them at the poly campout, and Morgan and Clark decided to go for a little walk and it was just me and Heather. I said, "Yeah, I'll watch her." So they go off and take their walk and I am making Heather a sandwich. They hadn't been gone for maybe five minutes when she just sits there and she looks at me and says, "James," and I said, "Yes, Heather?" and she said, "I love you." It was that moment that just knocked me out. And I said, "Well, I love you very much, too." We have a bond. I mean, she has said to me "you are like my other dad" or "you

are like my uncle." Every time I have been honored. . . . Brady is special because he is just four now, and Morgan and I got together when she was pregnant which is a story in and of itself. That is the closest, I am sure, I will ever come to being a dad. I was there through the entire pregnancy, before she even showed and then right through the birth. I was there rocking him to sleep, feeding him at three o'clock in the morning, changing diapers, making sure Morgan could sleep when Clark was down hanging out with my wife, I would be up here. I was here as much as I could be. And it was precious, and it was beautiful, and fantastic and that kid will have a place in my heart that I can't describe.

The fact that James (with Clark's help) made the effort to continue his relationship with Heather and Brady two years after breaking up with their mother attested to his enduring emotional connection with the children. While Brady was too young for me to interview at the time, I was able to ask his older sister, Heather, how she thought he felt about James. Heather responded:

Yeah, Brady really loved James, he was around all the time until like two years ago. I love James, too, I miss him now that he is not here nearly as much. But we get to see him sometimes. Not enough, but at least sometimes. Daddy takes us to see James, every other weekend or so we drive down to [a town about forty-five minutes away] to meet him for lunch and we play games and stuff. It's nice to see him, but it's not the same as when they were all together and we got to see him all the time, all all the time.

Clark, Morgan's husband and father to Heather and Brady, commented that he would routinely take the children to see James:

Oh yeah, we get to see him all the time. Either we drive down to [a town about forty-five minutes away] or he comes up here. Actually, usually we go down there, probably every other week or so. I actually get along with James better than Morgan does right now, so it makes sense for me to take Heather and Brady down to see him. I know the kids miss him a lot so I definitely put effort in to getting them together. I still like him, too, so it is nice for me to see him, though I don't think I would do it nearly as much if it weren't for the kids.

The fact that Clark maintained a more congenial relationship than Morgan did with James was characteristic of poly men who would help their children remain in contact with their wife or partner's former boyfriends. This happened most commonly among men who had not established a sexual relationship with each other, something I think allowed them to move more easily beyond the romantic stage of the relationship without the hurt feelings that their wives or girlfriends might harbor in relationship to their ex-lovers. It was also more common among men who respected each other and treated each other ethically—men who felt their female partner's ex-boyfriends had lied to them or mistreated their partners were much less likely to attempt to keep an ongoing relationship alive.

Even fathers connected by biology, legal ties, or long attentive association helped each other maintain contact with children after splitting up with the children's mothers. Patrick Wyss was part of the Wyss quad for fourteen years (and two years previously as part of a moresome) before moving out to live with Lucia and her son, Evan. Albert Wyss reported that, due to some logistical constraints and some personal taste:

> Neither Loretta nor Kiyowara arrange to see him [Patrick] regularly except for Kethry's school things, but he and I have lunch every Saturday with Kethry at Costco and then come home to watch British comedy TV. When I see Patrick it's because we are doing something with Kethry. I don't do things with him without Kethry. I have nothing massively against Patrick. I was not as emotionally charged about the whole thing when we were in the breakup. It was sad we could not get that to work out . . . Some of me hanging out with him is shared interest—we both like *Doctor Who* and BBC-type things that I have liked forever and am indoctrinating my child into, and Patrick is fond of as well. We like to watch the people shopping [at Costco] and comment on their fashion faux pas, or Patrick will talk about what is going on with his art installations and things from his art classes . . . it is enjoyable to go out and chat with Kethry and Patrick about what's going on. I see a little more about what Kethry is up to as well, because when she is chatting to Patrick she talks more about what happens in the role-playing game they both play. When she goes off to play I ask how it went and I get five- or ten-sentence summaries without a lot of detail, but when she talks to Patrick it is more involved because they both play.

At other points it was clear that Albert treasured his connection with Kethry and went out of his way to "meet her where she is," tailoring his schedule on vacation to fit Kethry's and wanting to know what she thought about and how she felt. Patrick similarly went to great lengths to see Kethry regularly, picking her up at the train station on her way home from school several days a week and playing role-playing games with her regularly. Patrick's connection with Kethry enhanced Albert's connection with Kethry because he got a glimpse of an expanded understanding of his daughter that he would otherwise not have seen. In other words, poly men can help each other deepen their relationships with their children and sustain contact in a way that appears to be quite difficult for serial-monogamous relationships that break up and in which are still overwhelmingly women who are single parents.[9]

It seemed in retrospect to the remaining triad that Patrick had slowly withdrawn from the quad, symbolized by his "stuff" being contained within his own bedroom—separate from the other three who shared a bed—and the outdoor workshop, but his stuff was notably absent from the other rooms, as evidenced by how little they changed when he moved out. Kiyowara had married Albert and Loretta independently, and the three had gotten rings together to symbolize their family connection, but Patrick did not marry Loretta or Albert, even though Patrick and Loretta had been sexually involved: The only nonpair was Patrick and Albert, both heterosexual men. Albert concluded: "We are still friends who see each other occasionally but no sexual interaction. Maybe it is easier to break up and still be friends if you weren't sexual, um. Hard to say, not enough data points."

Cohusbands

Far less familiar than co-wives or sister-wives, co-husbands (or even more awkwardly, brother-husbands) forge a new category for men rarely seen in any society. Men in poly families who share a relationship with the same woman defy the strict demands of mainstream masculinity that require "real" men to have exclusive sexual access to "their" women.[10] Far from being rivals, some men in poly families have deeply supportive, emotionally intimate relationships with each other. Characteristic of men who do "dude things" together, the Majek men collaborated on many major home repairs. Once when I arrived to interview they family, Clark, Nash, and James were all up on a scaffold out front, painting the house. Another time I found Nash and Clark laying paving stones to create a backyard walkway. Cooperating on work provided a familiar masculine territory for the men to establish and strengthen relationships, as well as making the house look great. Clark told me, "I'm thrilled to have the help, I learn a lot from these guys and it's too much work for one person. It's fun to hang out with them too, have a beer afterwards and check out the awesome stuff we did."

Summer and Zack Phoenix shared a house with Summer's lover Jared. Usually Zack and Summer shared the master bedroom and Jared slept in his own attached in-law apartment, but when Summer would travel out of town for work, sometimes the men would sleep together. Zack told me, "Sometimes when we are both really missing her we cuddle up in the big bed and talk about her or what happened during our day or whatever, and fall asleep. It's nice and comforting to have him there. We eat together and hang out, we're family." When Summer is gone, Jared and Zack keep each other company and avoid getting lonely.

Bjorn and Gene Tree have a similarly close relationship, enough so that when they are out in public together with their infant son Will they are routinely mistaken for a gay couple. Bjorn said:

> It's really funny to watch how people react to us in different combinations. When I'm with Leah and Will people don't really give us a second look except at the baby, but when I'm with Gene and Will I definitely get the feeling people think we are a couple by the way they react to us. We get more looks and more comments—usually smiles, sometimes "oh how cute," gay dads nodding to us at the playground. This is the Bay Area so gay couples are pretty common, so I guess in that way we kind of blend in, except that we're both straight. But we don't necessarily tell other people that, we just let them assume we are a couple with our son. Because we kind of are— definitely with our son at least, even if we're not a couple.

Sharing parenting, emotional intimacy, time, and their mutual love for Leah gave Gene and Bjorn an uncommon relationship that benefitted both of their lives. Outside of sports and activity-directed buddy relationships, mainstream men in the United States do not have a very wide range of emotional or relationship options,[11] and poly relationships provide men with new avenues to establish emotionally intimate, mutually supportive relationships with each other.

POLYAFFECTIVITY

All of these relationships we have discussed in this section of the chapter characterize polyaffectivity. Polyaffectivity differs from "regular" friendship in that the people involved see it as far more important than mainstream society usually views relationships that are not biologically, legally, or even sexually connected. People who love each other on that level hesitate to call themselves "just friends" because their friendships are among the most important relationships in their lives: the fact that they do not have sex does not mean they are "just" friends. Polyaffective relationships can develop the devotion and degree of seriousness that most people associate only with marriage (or at minimum an ongoing sexual relationship). Not all nonsexual relationships in poly situations are polyaffective: the participants must consider each other to be significant relationships to qualify as polyaffective. That is, people associated through poly relationships who are acquaintances or casual friends do not possess the emotional intimacy or expectation of mutual support that is present in polyaffective relationships. Polyaffectivity has a number of significant implications, as I'll discuss in greater detail later. It allows for a much wider variety of relationships and a far broader base of support than does a more conventional relationship that relies more heavily on the sometimes tenuous bonds of romantic love.

8

DIFFICULTIES IN POLYAMOROUS FAMILIES

While there are many advantages to a poly household, children and parents also describe a variety of disadvantages, including dealing with social stigma, children's emotional pain with the loss of a treasured adult after a breakup, household crowding, family complexities, and too much supervision. Importantly, the difficulties poly families face are the same difficulties facing other complex families in the United States today. Household crowding, partners breaking up, family drama, and even the most heinous family problem of child molestation are things that happen in nonpoly families as well. None of the problems the poly folks discussed were isolated to only people in polyamorous families.

STIGMA

In the discipline of sociology, the term *stigma* refers to "an attribute that is deeply discrediting,"[1] a personal characteristic that society has deemed undesirable and thus marks the stigmatized person as tainted or spoiled. Stigma always exists in social context and can change dramatically from one setting, historical era, or subculture to another. Fifty years ago, decorative tattoos on women were considered taboo—a scandalous rarity worthy of harsh whispers and social exclusion or pity. Now tattoos are so popular in mainstream U.S. culture that they have become commonplace, unremarkable on women in many age groups.

While stigma against people with tattoos has waned to a large extent, other stigmas such as those against people of color or sexual minorities prove more durable. If increased public acceptance of same-sex marriage and neutral or positive media portrayals of same-sex relationships are any indication, mainstream public opinion in the United States appears to be shifting toward greater acceptance of people perceived as gay, lesbian, or (to a somewhat lesser extent) transgendered. Even so, homophobia, sexual prejudice, and sex negativity—all reciprocal symptoms and causes of stigma against sexual minorities—remain important social forces. Coming out or being exposed as a sexual minority can still result in alienation from family and friends,[2] physical attack or harassment,[3] loss of a job or custody of a child,[4] public degradation, and incarceration.[5]

One of the primary disadvantages facing poly families is the stigma associated with being sexual minorities. I have found that their social privileges and a comparatively low level of public awareness that allows/forces poly people to remain invisible provides mainstream polyamorists some protection from the effects of stigma. Nonetheless, poly families experience and fear a variety of stigma-related issues including social rejection, fear that their children will be negatively affected, their children's experiences of stigma, institutional vulnerability resulting from stigma, and the leverage that vulnerability gives disgruntled teens.

Social Rejection

While Melody Lupine's triad with Cristof and Quentin had never been fully embraced by portions of their social circle, even those who had accepted the triad became increasingly intolerant when Melody intentionally became pregnant with Quentin's child while still married to Cristof. Melody remembered that friends expressed discomfort and

> judgments, how could you do that, it's immoral and you know, how could you do that to Cristof. And that baby's gonna grow up being so confused. They thought it was worse than cheating, that you have a baby with someone else while you're married to somebody was just beyond, just unfathomable to people. And even some polyamorous people were pretty judgmental about it. . . .

Breaking such an important norm as bearing solely the husband's children while married was more than some of the Lupines' associates would tolerate, and they rejected Melody and her family. While the triad and their children paid for their nonconformity, there were some advantages as well. It gave Melody the opportunity to have the third child she had wanted (which Cristof did not wish to father), and Quentin a "second chance" at parenting now that his older children were grown.

Rejection from Family Members

Poly people can lose not only friends but relationships with family members as well. Baldwin Omni, a middle-class white man in his early sixties, experienced the social backlash of stigma when his adult children Rosaline and Wade, wife Nadia, and Nadia's extended family rejected him for becoming polyamorous. At our initial interview, Baldwin identified himself as being in a poly/mono relationship, albeit "not the typical one." He continued:

> From 1974 to 1980 my wife and I had an open marriage in the sense that we sometimes played with others, always with each other's knowledge, sometimes in their presence, occasionally with their participation. We didn't really "date"; these were generally people we or one of us already knew and were curious about. It wasn't equivalent to poly, cause amory wasn't part of the equation. Any intimate encounters did not affect the underlying friendships and make them more of a relationship. We also attended a few swinging parties and decided that was too casual for us.

Then in 1980, when pregnant with their first child, Baldwin said that Nadia: "became much more conservative, said 'I don't want to do this any more, I feel it's wrong' and so I became totally mono for twenty-six years." Baldwin, deeply dismayed about the turn of events, reported that "had she not been pregnant I might have left her." Nadia had a son they named Wade, and three years later Baldwin and Nadia had a daughter named Rosaline, and they appeared for all intents and purposes as a conventional family.

Baldwin reported that "the kids and I got along great when they were little," but as they aged Nadia and Baldwin disagreed on how to discipline the children and they eventually "solidified into dad as the enforcer and mom as the nurturer." Further alienating Baldwin from the children, he had what he described as the "job from hell" and "came home frustrated and angry every day. The kids would hear the front door and go hide in their rooms, deal with me as little as possible. There was also a lot of frustration and resentment over Nadia's increasing involvement in her church." This left what Baldwin characterized as "a lot of baggage" in his relationship with his children, "predisposing them to think poorly of me in relationship to the poly," although he admitted, "I definitely left something to be desired as a father."

In 2006, Nadia initiated what Baldwin termed a "remarkable conversation" in which she

> thanked me for my years of loving, faithful partnership and said that she felt somewhat guilty for "inhibiting who you have always been" . . . she said, "I changed but you didn't, I never expected you to follow my new standards of morality, but I was glad you did." Still, it bothered her that it inhibited me. She also recognized that anything else that happened back in the old days didn't affect my commitment to her then, and offered that if I wanted to have some discreet and safe adventures that would be OK, but she would prefer not to know about them at all.

Baldwin "took her up on the offer" and began a series of forays into the dating world, making sure to be discreet and careful of sexually transmitted infections. Dating new people brought new experiences, and Baldwin experienced significant personal growth and some sexual adventures.

Eventually Baldwin established a relationship with Abigail and began seeing her once a week. Nadia oscillated between trying to accept his relationships and feeling terrible about them. At one point Nadia encouraged Baldwin to take one of his dates to their timeshare condo at Lake Tahoe and that he should "be sure to take her to our favorite romantic bistro on a pier overlooking the lake for dinner. I'd say that was pretty compersive!" Alternately, Baldwin thought Nadia began to drink more and was quite upset with him regularly, eventually saying that she accepted and allowed but did not approve of my relationships. From her Christian faith perspective, poly is wrong. I pointed out that I have accepted, even grown to support her participation in a faith practice that I feel is wrong, because of how much it's a part of her life and how much it nourishes her. There's also the issue that she has been having an intimate poly relationship with Jesus Christ for the last thirty years and when she goes away for a weekend or a week or whatever for a church retreat or conference its like going away with her lover—except that there isn't physical sex, but it might even be more intimate than that. She bristled, and said sharply that she was "just exercising her faith." Oh really? Every morning she would wake up one-half hour before my alarm went off and go upstairs to the den to pray out loud and "be with The Lord." When she came down, she brought me a mug of coffee in bed. I sometimes asked, "May I please have a hug to reconnect with you after you've been with Him?," but she would just sit up in bed and read a tract published by her church . . . She's also nervous about the social issue, if her friends or family find out that her husband is basically having an ongoing affair with another woman with her consent, how will they judge her for allowing that?

Although Baldwin had been "excruciatingly discreet," eventually his children found out that he was having polyamorous relationships. Baldwin reported that, when he took a date on an overnight trip to a hot springs, Rosaline asked where he was and Nadia

outed me, saying I was there with this woman. Nadia thought Rosaline would be OK. Nope. She totally disapproved, and wondered how Mom could tolerate being with "such a man." Rosaline told Wade, who actually came over and wanted to physically pummel me, but his mother stopped him at the door. She told him it was consensual; he could not accept that. He said to his mother that I am dead to him because of what I "did to her." Nadia told him we had an agreement and it was consensual, but it had no impact. Nor did the fact that our wedding vows, which we wrote to deliberately exclude the "forsaking all others" part, and also did not include the "til death do us part."

Baldwin's children began to "harass their mother, putting a lot of pressure on Mom to leave me because of the poly. She tried to tell them that we have a non-typical relationship, but it didn't matter. They

acted like Dad was pressuring Mom into something and she caved in."
Later, Baldwin mentioned that "while Nadia would prefer it was not
happening, she has consented to it voluntarily."

Over two years Baldwin continued dating, having a serious relationship with Abigail and less serious relationships with several other wom-
en. Baldwin said that Nadia was

> struggling with it, feeling somewhat jealous, trying to handle it. She
> is intellectually OK with it, but emotionally it's very difficult, particu-
> larly the societal mores and her church's belief that anything like
> poly is wrong, our kids' disapproval, and some "primal jealousy" as
> she calls it. Still, she knows I am committed to her/us, and she said
> she has to handle it somehow as neither of us wants to split.

While Nadia struggled with her angst over Baldwin's polyamorous
relationships, things went from bad to worse in Baldwin's relationships
with his children, until neither child would speak to him or come over
to their parents' house if Baldwin was home. Family holidays became
tense, and Baldwin reported that

> I went to Thanksgiving with Nadia at my sister-in-law's, and both
> kids were there. Not one word was spoken between us. About a week
> before Wade outed me to Nadia's cousin, who usually has a Thanks-
> giving dessert and coffee thing. Wade explained why he was so upset
> and refused to talk to me, and Nadia's cousin sent a message back
> through Wade to Nadia and me that I was uninvited from the
> Thanksgiving dessert party. I don't know what Wade said, but I can
> be sure it wasn't flattering. He is the one who told Nadia "poly is just
> Dad's bullshit intellectual justification for fucking around."

Even with all of his assertions that Nadia was allowing him to be polyamorous voluntarily, by December she decided that she could not tolerate the relationship style.

> She said poly just wasn't working for her. She initially reserved the
> right to change her mind. It destroyed my relationship with both kids
> and caused a strain on Nadia. She said she wants me to move out.
> This is all being handled very amicably, and one evening I was crying
> and saying I was sorry, and Nadia said, "For what, being who you
> have always been?" Then another night she was sobbing in the car,

and said, "I'm really going to miss you, but this is the only way for both of us." We are hoping that once we are no longer living in a minefield, having the same fight over and over for three decades, we can be friends. So part of me is feeling like "bad dog, bad dog!" and I'm being exiled from the home I've lived in for twenty-seven years, but most of the time I feel like I'm being given the freedom to be fully myself and happier than I have ever been.

Baldwin experienced significant social censure for his engagement in polyamorous relationships, and while he gained a sense of freedom and joy, it came at the expense of his relationships with his wife and children. Although so many marriages break up after years when the husband wants to experiment sexually with younger women that it has become cliché, few of them do so with the honesty and integrity that Baldwin and Nadia brought to bear on the end of their marriage.

POTENTIAL TO INFLICT PAIN ON CHILDREN

Parents in poly families were painfully aware that their children have or may face the difficult chore of managing the stigma of their parents' unconventional relationships, and some parents expressed remorse about the pain their relationships have caused their children. Joya Starr recounted her sadness over the challenges her polyamorous lifestyle created for her then six-year-old son Gideon, when

> he started going to school and they were asking "Who's your mommy, who's your daddy?" And he's able to identify us biologically without a problem. But for him it felt like—why are they only asking about those people? Like those are the only important people? . . . Now he knows this information about mom being poly and whatnot can actually really scare and freak people out. And having him be so young and having to manage that amount of responsibility for how adults and other kids relate to him, I can sometimes feel regret . . . And I wish that I was in a more stable trio for him so that he had this solid place to come from instead of like this multiple relating, my marriage didn't work kind of thing.

While Joya was keenly aware of the difficulty her son faced in relation to her polyamorous lifestyle, true to what she saw as her polyamorous nature, her ideal solution was a more stable poly family, rather than a monogamous one.

Melody Lupine similarly reported a deep conflict between her role as editor of a polyamorous magazine and a parent of children who wished to

> be normal. The website needs some new pictures and I am the logical choice, with my kids even better for the site. But for my kids? Definitely not! I would never ask them to put their pictures on the web—I am not sure if I can even put my own picture on the website. What if one of their friend's parents sees it and then it hurts my kids somehow? That would be terrible! I have to walk a fine line, decide each time to come out or not depending on the impact on my kids.

In weighing the needs of the magazine versus the needs of her family, Melody prioritized her children's perceived emotional well-being and used a picture of herself alone.

Children's Experiences of Stigma

Children in poly families were also aware of the potential for stigma, and occasionally they had direct experiences of it. While Zoe Hadaway had not experienced negative reactions to coming out as being a member of a poly family, she imagined that she would and was thus extremely careful about those with whom she discussed her family. "The disadvantage socially is, you don't know how people are going to react until after you tell them. And that, their reaction, is how they feel about that problem—it makes or breaks the decision of whether or not to tell them." Silas Hadaway reported that he did not often invite his friends over after school because he was reluctant to explain the multiple adults living in his household: "I guess it kind of keeps me from having friends, sometimes, but I am kinda shy anyway, and even before we all moved in I didn't have friends over all the time, or very much at all."

Overall, the children I spoke with did not report experiencing many significant experiences of stigma. There are at least three explanations for this relative dearth of experiences of stigma. First, this could be because of the people who chose to volunteer for the research and their generally optimistic view of polyamorous families. Second, the race and class privileges that provide many of these children with social advantages may shield them from some of the effects of stigma. Third, the fact that poly families are still relatively unknown makes them more difficult to recognize and can protect them from the stigma of being recognizable sexual minorities.

Family Vulnerability

People in poly families were also aware that the stigma of being a sexual minority made them more vulnerable to accusations of poor parenting or questionable family situations from relatives, neighbors, teachers, and Child Protective Services (CPS, sometimes called Division of Family and Children Services or DFCS) officials. Social stigma places polyamorists at a disadvantage, because disclosure or discovery of what Goffman would call their "discrediting status" can give a boss, angry teenager, or extended family member leverage to use against the poly person. In some cases, the presence of polyamorous relationships made interaction with CPS officials even more frightening for parents who had come to the authorities' attention for other, nonpoly reasons. Evelyn Coach remembered the pain she felt when her daughter, Annabelle—six years old at the time, struggling with urinary tract infections due to an undiagnosed physical anomaly, and recently diagnosed with ADHD—was taken in to protective custody on a Friday afternoon before a three-day weekend.

> Our child was summarily removed from our care without question and placed in foster care. I was told nothing, other than that I could bring her medications and a toy or anything else she might need. We had no idea what the source of the issue was, whether there was *real* abuse that had happened—like at the hands of a stranger or someone in the neighborhood—or whether someone had misconstrued our [poly] lifestyle in some way. On Tuesday when I spoke with someone by phone, they told me that the source of the call was someone at school and that the quick action was because they suspected my husband Mark of sexually abusing our daughter. At least then we could relax about whether something had actually happened to Annabelle! But now we had to be prepared for the possibility of Mark facing a court battle to somehow prove his innocence. It took them until Wednesday to have someone talk directly to Annabelle, at

which time they immediately determined that no, she was obviously NOT an abused child.

By Thursday social services allowed the Coachs to come in and explain themselves, and the social worker "lectured [us] for our in-house nudism." The social worker was "at least somewhat understanding of some of our choices" and explained that Annabelle had made a comment to a teacher that her father "played doctor to her," by which Annabelle meant that Mark had put ointment on her rash. Evelyn said that "the officials had put together that comment, her toileting issues, and her ADHD issues, made some assumptions about her responses to questions like 'did he touch you down there?' and decided that she fit the profile of an abused child" and removed her from the Coach's custody.

Annabelle's removal from her parents not only traumatized all three of them significantly but also interfered with her schooling and new medication. Most significantly, it singled Annabelle out from her peers at school and created a lasting tension and fear in the Coach household.

> The incident has colored our family ever since. Mark took to wearing clothing around the house, albeit resentfully. We changed the policies on a large event we host, to separate kids from nudity, and keeping even our own child off site during the part allowing adult, nonsexual nudity. We lived in fear of the next time someone would report us for something out of ignorance. My husband became depressed and anxious. My own depression and anxiety worsened. And my daughter, formerly bold and uninhibited, developed social anxiety with strangers, which persists to this day.

The Coachs dealt with the trauma by becoming even more "out" as polyamorous activists, offering public education to "help ensure that others would not need to go through the same terror and fear of being 'outed' or misunderstood for making a choice to have more loving adults present in their lives, and the lives of their children." While Evelyn is grateful for the perspective the experience provided and the insight it gave her into other's experiences, the thought of that episode still sickens her even years later. "I wouldn't wish that experience on my own worst enemy."

Evelyn, Annabelle, and Mark were all traumatized by the incident. Annabelle referred hesitantly to the episode in an interview when she was eleven years old but was reluctant to discuss it further:

Elisabeth: Do people in your school know that your parents are poly? No? Why not?

Annabelle: Kind of . . . not something to talk about at school.

Elisabeth: How come?

Annabelle: [pause, then in a low voice] It's just not really [pause] something to talk about at school.

Elisabeth: So who can you talk about it with?

Annabelle: The cat. (laughter)

Evelyn: [to Annabelle] It's okay to tell her the stuff that happened that we had to be a little more close-mouthed about it. No? OK.

Elisabeth: We'll talk about something else then. So you have friends in the Pagan community who know you're poly. Are some of them poly too?

It was obvious from Annabelle's demeanor that she was still uncomfortable discussing it, and she seemed nervous remembering what had happened five years earlier. Clearly, the experience had been negative for her.

While Mark and Evelyn were able to regain custody of Annabelle in less than a week, Warren Bien's three daughters Rebecca, Callie, and Macy were placed in foster care when they were removed from their mother Julie's house and lived at a foster home for months before Warren was able to regain custody of the children. Warren and Julie married in the early 1990s and became polyamorous almost immediately. Over the years they had two daughters—Rebecca and Callie—and dated a variety of people. Eventually Julie established a serious relationship with Andrew, a friend of the family who had moved to the area to find a job. Warren said that Andrew was "interested in doing family things with us, since he did not have any relatives in the area. He started spending more time with us, and he and Julie developed an interest in each other." In 2000 Andrew moved in with Julie, Warren, and the girls, and Andrew and Julie later had a daughter named Macy who Warren also considered his daughter. Warren reported that

> at first it went well, and after a while I also had Estella, one of my partners, move in and the family moved together to a different state. At that point it started to involve other things besides poly. My oldest daughter said that her now stepfather Andrew started molesting her in 2002. That lasted for about three years, and I was not aware of it at the time . . . In late 2005 I decided my marriage was not salvageable; Julie and I had not communicated about anything but child care in two years. I did not feel I was important to her beyond a paycheck and I did not think that was going to change, so I moved out with Estella and her husband, Devon. Julie has since become extremely emotionally and financially dependent on Andrew. Then, in 2008, Estella and Rebecca were talking about the time we all lived together and Rebecca tells Estella that Andrew had molested her during that time. On her ninth birthday Andrew took Rebecca out to a movie and stopped at a truckers' motel on the way back and had oral sex with her. Rebecca is not sure how many times it happened over the next three years, but there were times when the two of them would go out on the property of our forty-acre wooded lot and there were other occasions when he would go into her bedroom at night.

Elisabeth: Why didn't she say anything at the time?

Warren: Andrew made quite an effort to ensure that she enjoyed the experience so she was not sure if it qualified as rape. She didn't know who should could talk to that would believe her and do something about it. Even at that point, her mother was getting more and more dependent on Andrew, and I spent a lot more time out of the house at work than I did at home so I was there but not as much of the time as I probably should have been. Most of the time that I was there and awake the girls were at school. At one point I was working sixteen-hour days.

Elisabeth: So what happened when Rebecca told Estella?

Warren: Estella called me at work and asked me to come home. When Rebecca told me what happened, I immediately called the sheriff's office and they sent a deputy out to take her statement that evening and I called the DFACS hotline soon after he left. At this time Estella and I were living with her husband, Devon, and Andrew and Julie were living in the same house that we had moved out of, maybe twenty or twenty-five minutes away. Callie lived with Julie and had regular visits with me, and Rebecca had been living with me since July of 2007 when I had moved from an apartment to a house that was large enough for her to have a bedroom. Macy was living with her mom [Julie].

Elisabeth: What did you do after the whole story came out?

Warren: I believed Rebecca and took action. I called Julie and said I wanted custody of Callie as well, and at first it seemed as though she was going to be reasonable about it . . . but over the course of the next week she decided that Rebecca was not telling the truth, which absolutely thrilled Rebecca [sarcastically]. My opinion is that Julie can't afford emotionally or financially to believe that her husband is a child molester.

Elisabeth: How has that worked out with the courts?

Warren: In early July 2008 the DCS asked that all three of the girls be placed in safe custody while they investigated what was going on in both households. That is still ongoing [as of April 2009]. Julie has limited supervised visitation with the two younger girls, without her husband who has been barred from all contact with any of the kids, and Julie has also been barred from visiting with Rebecca. Rebecca has expressed some interest in seeing her mom, but Rebecca's therapist thinks it would be bad for her to see her mom . . . I have had much more extensive visitation in my home, unsupervised, with all three girls, since November, which was a pleasant surprise. That has gone very well and the girls are happy to be here on the weekends and enjoy spending time with me . . . They say they want to come live with me all the time . . . I think it is very likely that the older two girls at least will be living here at the end of the school year. Julie is still living with someone who is on trial for the rape of a child, so the youngest daughter will probably not move back in with her mom. The judge lets her come over here on the weekends, so she might be able to come when the older girls move back in as well. I want her to move in with me with the other two, I think of her as my daughter and she calls me her papa bear.

Warren said his divorce had nothing to do with polyamory, that he and Julie had communication issues that predated their polyamorous relationships. The transition from a household of five adults and three children to two separate households had been a challenge for everyone, but the adults remained unaware of Andrew's molestation of Rebecca that had already occurred. Once the information came out, Warren asked Callie about possible molestation, and she had responded that "Andrew had never touched her."

In an effort to "encourage the courts to place the kids with me," Warren and his lawyer decided that he should live separately from Estella and Devon so "the court was not looking at a poly household." Having to separate from his lover Estella and her husband Devon, whom Warren loved like a brother, was devastating to Warren at a time when he needed his support system around him. Warren said that the court case had "interfered with my relationships but not ended them."

When I asked why the girls went into foster care and were not placed with him in the first place, Warren responded:

> I briefly had custody of Callie but while the hearing was going on to determine if temporary custody should be continued or not, Julie made some allegations in the courtroom specifically regarding Devon. She said that she believed that Rebecca had been molested, but she did not believe that it was her husband that was doing it, and while she did not say so specifically it was clear she was implying that it had been Devon. The judge said that he was not in a position to determine the truth of that matter, so instead of placing the kids in either household where they may or may not be at risk, he was going to place them elsewhere . . . I am pretty sure I would have gotten the kids right away if I had not been poly.
>
> Elisabeth: Do you think the molestation would not have happened if your family had not been poly?
>
> Warren: I don't think that is accurate. Whether Julie and I had been sexually open before it occurred or not, we still would have had other friends and while it might have been more difficult for Andrew to

have access to my daughter if he had not been in a sexual relationship with Julie, I am fairly certain he still would have been a friend of the family and I think it is likely that he would have had access to her [Rebecca] anyway. So he [Andrew] caused the molestation, not polyamory.

Child molestation has in recent years been revealed to be a major social issue, so unfortunately widespread that it is not confined only to sexual minorities, people with unconventional lifestyles, or children who attend Catholic churches. Even so, it was extremely disadvantageous to this child in this poly family who was molested by one of her parent's partners—a terrible turn of events no parent would want to subject their children to.

Teenagers Have Leverage Against Poly Parents

Because authorities can be suspicious of anything out of the ordinary, the stigma of being in an unconventional family can make some poly parents vulnerable to attempted blackmail from disgruntled teenagers. The Holstrom family was composed of Billy and Megan, a married couple with a daughter, Ariel, of their union; a son, Nolan, from Megan's previous marriage; and a son, Simon, from Billy's previous marriage; Jack (Megan's partner); Sabine (Billy's partner); and Tad (Sabine's husband). Things were going along smoothly until Nolan "blew his stack," as Billy reported. Nolan had run into Rex, his biological father, while visiting relatives in another state, and Billy said that Nolan

used it as ammunition against us when he got back. Ammunition for anything he could use to hurt his mother [Megan]. We never found out why he wanted to hurt her before he got us kicked out of family therapy. He thinks we kept him from his dad even though his dad was in the federal penitentiary in jail for selling firearms to an undercover agent . . . He was in jail for . . . over half of Nolan's life when Nolan found him.

In an attempt to interrupt a negative behavior cycle in which Nolan was "being ugly and violent, getting in trouble at school, hanging with the wrong crowd," Megan had "sent him [Nolan] away from that element to change his scene." Unfortunately, taking a break from the "wrong crowd" did not significantly alter Nolan's behavior, and Billy reported that when Nolan returned:

> We knew something was up but we didn't know what. He caused a big scene, decided he was going to be big and bad and take a swing at me so I had him arrested for assault, terroristic threats, and cruelty to children because all of this happened in front of Ariel. He spent the night in jail and did an arraignment the next morning, and this is where poly enters the story. Through all of this we had tried to fix it on our own; we went to family therapy but he would not go to individual counseling, he was not in it to fix whatever problem there was. So before we go into the courtroom the public defender asks if there is anything we need to say but once we get in the courtroom and the judge sentences him [Nolan] to eighteen months supervised, so then the judge asks, "What is this I hear about you having someone extra in your relationship? Don't you know that adultery is against the law?" I [Billy] said that it was not illegal to love more than one person, and the judge said, "Adultery is illegal in [this state]!" and he tells us we have to go to counseling and we will be investigated by DFACS and we need to reevaluate our relationship choices to make sure we are doing what is best for our family. So instead of putting the responsibility on Nolan for his own behavior, the cause was legally shifted to us where we were the bad guys.

Over the next several months the family was under DFACS surveillance, with home visits and case managers visiting Ariel at school. Billy reported telling the DFACS case manager:

> Anything that happens in our bedroom stays there. Have you ever had a sleepover? That is about how much the kids get to see, everything beyond that happens in the bedroom. That was good, she seemed to understand poly . . . So the case went on and she interviewed us, Jack, Megan, Megan's mom, and some of Ariel's teachers. After about a month we had not heard anything so we called her and asked what was happening. She said, "You didn't hear? I certified you as a perfectly functioning family and Nolan sounds like he needs to work on himself." It turns out Nolan got a girl pregnant, lied to us and lied to her, and then she lied and said she lost the baby even though she was still pregnant. We didn't know any of this until we went to court, and that's when it all fell into place what Nolan's

problem had been—he'd gotten somebody pregnant and didn't know how to talk to us so he was weird and angry.

While the DFACS case manager appeared to understand the polyamorous dynamic in the Holstrom family, Nolan's probation officer took a decidedly different approach to the family. Billy reported:

The juvenile justice system on the whole has a negative attitude toward poly or any alternative lifestyle. The probation officer would say things like "the way you people are," or "the lifestyle that you participate in is not normal, that is not a normal household." . . . We didn't hide anything, and it became apparent that because we were different, she judged us negatively . . . Now Nolan lives with a friend whose mom is unemployed, in the middle of a divorce, has five teenagers, but his probation officer thinks that is still a better place for him than what she called "THAT household with all that STUFF going on." Nolan swears up and down that all of his problems are because we are poly, that he just can't live that way. I told him you don't have to live that way, you just have to accept people who are different from you. We thought we had raised an open-minded, accepting child only to have it blow up in our faces. Our other son has no problems at all with it; he would go to the moon and back for us. He hasn't said anything about it; he sees nothing wrong with people living their lives the way they want to live. Not his cup of tea right now, but whatever we do is fine with him . . . and it is not even like Jack lives with us, he lives several hours away in [a city] and comes up to visit two or three weekends a month. That is the other thing that puzzled us, with Jack not being here all the time, he [Nolan] was always angry. If it was really about the poly, then why be so angry all the time and not just when we are doing poly activities? Now we only hear from Nolan when he needs money, and I told him to call his dad for that because his dad owes him a quarter of a million dollars in back child support he never paid. Nolan said that was not fair, and I said we don't have any money so ask your bio dad.

Frustrated with their son's refusal to take responsibility for himself and angry at the juvenile justice system that judged them so harshly, Billy and Megan felt the impacts of institutional stigma that aggravated their existing family problems.

After the investigation ended the Holstrom family "did not hear a peep from DFACS since," and Billy and Megan began to relax because it appeared DFACS would not remove their youngest child, Ariel, from the home. Ariel's teachers and social support circle all reported to DFACS that Ariel was doing fine and the Holstrom family seemed to be free of further surveillance. Even so, Billy reported:

> This actually has Megan and I talking about a legal divorce, though there is no statute of limitations on adultery. If we divorce it would prevent anything like this from happening again because if we were divorced we would no longer be committing the crime of adultery in [this state]. We would be committing fornication and cohabitation, bigamous cohabitation where two people who are assumed to be married living in the same house but having sexual relations with other people. The third party can also be charged with adultery and bigamy in [this state] . . . At this point they could also go after Jack, who lives in [a neighboring state] and comes to visit regularly. The penalties are different for each crime and in each state. In [Billy and Megan's home state] you can be prosecuted on a felony level for bigamous cohabitation, but fornication and regular cohabitation are misdemeanors if I remember correctly . . . We [Billy and Megan] would divorce only as a legal protective measure, not because we are unhappy together. More of an annulment than a divorce, I guess.

In order to protect their family from the legal ramifications of non-monogamy, Billy and Megan felt they had to dissolve their legal marriage—something other poly families have reported as well. In their case, outdated laws against fornication, adultery, and cohabitation selectively enforced against polyamorists and other sexual minorities—but not generally applied to heterosexual "vanilla" relationships—made Billy and Megan Holstrom more vulnerable to their teenage son's angst and attempts at manipulation. This level of vulnerability to authorities that might misunderstand or misjudge poly families based on the stigma against sexual nonconformists has been disadvantageous for polyamorists and other sexual minorities.

CHILDREN BECOME ATTACHED TO PARTNERS WHO LEAVE

While the presence of numerous adults attending to children in polyamorous families may provide an atmosphere of love and caring, it also sets the stage for children to become attached to adults who are related to them through the potentially tenuous bonds of a polyamorous relationship. Many parents reported their children's attachment to partners who eventually left the relationship, much to the children's chagrin. Joya Starr remembered her son Gideon's misery after the departure of one of her boyfriends, a man who had been the boy's treasured friend, and how Gideon had asked her, "I know why you guys are breaking up, but why does he have to break up with me too?"

Shelly and Sven Heartland formed a triad with Adam when their daughter Alice was a small child, and Alice became very attached to Adam over time. Even though he did not live with them, Adam spent almost all of his free time with the Heartlands and became quite close to the whole family. When Adam broke up with Shelly and Sven, Alice was heartbroken. Shelly reported that, even two or three years later:

> Alice will still call him and leave him messages and then when he doesn't call back that doesn't make her very happy 'cause when, she doesn't really understand why, even though he's not around any more, why he won't kind of respond to her, and he's pretty much cut off all ties with her.

While the entire family mentioned missing Adam at one point or another in their interviews, it seemed to be especially poignant for Alice, who loved Adam as a father.

Alice's sister Elise said she noticed a difference in Alice after Adam left and when Rich, Sven's new boyfriend, arrived. Elise said:

> Like when Richie came in to the picture and I was like talking to Alice about it, 'cause I don't know if she totally understands everything, and I was just like "Hey, how do you like Rich and stuff?" and she was like "He's no Adam." So she is still like totally attached to him [Adam] and stuff.

Similar to Alice, Cole related his pain at missing his parent's former girlfriend Bettina:

> The only thing I really regret is that, now that Bettina's gone, and her kids, that was the hard part. Just having them leave. Because they were such a huge influence in my life. I wasn't always regretting them, a lot of times they were really helpful. They got me out of a lot

of situations, and I learned a lot from the kids. . . I miss her [Bettina]
a great deal. And I wish I could see her more but she's moved away. I
wish I could just take her out to lunch, see how she's doing. . . I
always thought she would be here to help me through high school,
but she's not. I made it through my first year without her, and, well,
um, but I think about her a lot. I really miss her.

Cole said that he missed not only Bettina, his parents' ex-girlfriend,
but also her children, with whom he had established friendships bordering at some points on sibling relationships. He found it especially
painful when Bettina did not attend his bar mitzvah, an important rite
of passage for young Jewish men who spend years preparing to be
called to recite portions of the Torah and are then ushered into religious adulthood.

Cole: She wanted to come to my bar mitzvah. I always knew I would
have one, and I always knew she would be there. I thought my
parents had sent an invite, but it turns out they didn't. And I never
confronted my parents, they never found out I was angry. I asked her
what happened and she said I never got an invite, when was it, how
was it kind of thing, you know, a few days after my bar mitzvah. And
I realized she wasn't there, and after that, I never really talked to her,
pretty much after that.

Elisabeth: Why did you stop talking to her after that?

Cole: I guess maybe part of it was that I got a cue from my parents
that, maybe it was a false cue, but again I got a feeling from my
parents that they didn't want me talking to her. That they didn't want
me as part of her, as part of my life any more. I don't think that's
what happened, I just think that they honestly forgot or that, you
know, maybe there was some harsh breakup feelings but I don't
think they have them now.

Two years later, Cole asked his parents about failing to invite Bettina to
the bar mitzvah, and they assured him it had been an oversight, that if
he had wanted her to come he should have told them.

While some of the children I interviewed keenly missed beloved
adults who had exited their parents' lives, many of them did not. For
instance, Zane did not feel damaged by his parents' partners leaving.

I mean, I liked a lot of them, I was friends with them, but I was so used to them not being permanent that it was fine. I was glad I met them and I was happy to spend time with them but it was never like, I never thought too much about it. It was not a big deal. One specifically I remember, I was in sixth grade or something, I'd do a bunch with them. I'd skateboard with them, I'd ski with them, it was kind of just like an older friend. It wasn't that big of a deal that he left, I wasn't too bummed out. Just someone to hang out with, I guess. They were on and off again for a really long time, I can't even remember the time span. It was like pretty long, but it was always on and off. And he's still a friend, he's still around sometimes. He's cool, I like him. It wasn't like I avoided being friends with them or anything, I just kind of eventually warmed up to him. Like I said, it never was really that big of a deal. I don't know why, it never really crossed my mind as a bad thing that they were leaving.

Like Zane, many others did not see their parents' partners exit on a permanent basis but rather retained friendly contact with the family over time.

Partners could also become attached to children, and then feel upset when the relationship with the parents dissolved and the partner no longer spent as much time with the child of their former partners. When Kristine broke up with Mark and Evelyn, she missed their daughter, Annabelle, keenly.

While I was with Evelyn and Mark, there was a lot of love and it rips me apart to have had to walk away from Annabel. She became a priority for me, and often I spent more time with her than either of her parents. . . I remember weeks taking care of her [Annabelle], helping her with her homework, spending time with her. One time I was down with food poisoning, and I still spent an hour-and-a-half brushing out her hair of knots and tangles.

While Kristine felt loved when she was with the Coach family and thought that Evelyn and Mark were "extremely loving parents, really devoted to their daughters," Kristine was not sure that polyamory was a positive thing for the children or the family as a whole.

But I don't honestly believe that either Annabel or Martine benefited from Evelyn and Mark being poly, other than more adults riding herd on Annabel. Would they have benefited from them being monogamous? I don't know the marriage would have lasted as long, but there might have been fewer distractions.

I was unable to talk with Martine, but Annabelle reported to me that she felt she had gained numerous advantages from being in a poly family and did not identify the disadvantages Kristine found so distracting.

In this instance with the Coach family, the complexity of the adult relationships did not appear to translate to complexity in the child's relationship. In other cases, children see adult relationships in a worse light than do the adults engaged in them. Elise Heartland watched her mother

> go through hell with Adam. I mean you guys loved each other and obviously it was a good thing for you in some ways, but from where I stood it looked like a lot of pain.
>
> Shelly: But you didn't see us all the time, there are whole parts of the relationship you didn't see.
>
> Elise: Of course. But the parts I did see, it looked like a lot of pain and work for not that much fun for you. Sven seemed to do better with it, but Adam loved him that way too. I couldn't handle that, that would piss me off. There is no way, I need more attention than that. Like if I was with somebody and he was with somebody else I would be like really annoyed, that I'm going to go get another boyfriend.
>
> Shelly: I wasn't really angry with Adam, that was just the way it was.

Like everything else, the disadvantages and complexities have widely varying impacts on different members of the family, each can view the situation quite differently, and the same member can shift views over time.

Cole Cypress had a complex relationship with polyamory, and found it both good and bad at different times and in different ways. In chapter 7 Cole discussed taking the pocket knives to school and getting in trouble, and I asked him about how, if at all, that related to his family.

Elisabeth: When you were having your episode of being very angry and upset, acting up at school with the knives and stuff, did that have anything to do with polyamory?

Cole: I'm sure it did. I'm sure then was probably one of my bigger episodes of just like, you guys forced your lifestyle upon me, I never had any real friends because of you. And I just had a lot of hatred and that was the perfect scapegoat. Polyamory. I wasn't getting good grades and uh, there was also an issue with me swearing in school, cause this is of course a private school. And whenever my teachers ask me why I swear so much I would always always blame Bettina's son Caz . . .

Elisabeth: So you mentioned that you felt like you never had any friends because your parents were polyamorous?

Cole: I never, I feel like I never had any friends—I felt like I never had any friends just because I couldn't explain it to them. I couldn't really open up to them. It was 'cause of polyamory. I felt like all of my life was centered, centered around it now, and if I ever told the story about my life it would involve somebody from the poly community and I'd have to go into a whole explanation of polyamory and so I stayed away from people.

Elisabeth: Was that painful?

Cole: Yes. It was, yeah, yeah. It was extraordinarily painful just to (breathes deeply) just to live a life uh, you know, without friends. Uh, I would always, I was like a pariah, or an outcast in a class of forty-seven students or so.

Elisabeth: Specifically because of the polyamory?

Cole: Well, I felt that way. It wasn't though. Because I was acting out and because nobody wanted to be my friend. I wouldn't talk to people, I would swear and get in trouble and talk back to teachers, I didn't get good grades. I didn't like people that much. People didn't like me.

Elisabeth: Because you felt different?

Cole: Yeah.

Elisabeth: And you acted different? And the difference was based in the polyamory?

Cole: Yeah, it was based on that and just, you know, trying to live up to Caz, live up to his behavior.

Elisabeth: So that was a big factor.

Cole: Yeah, pretty much.

Elisabeth: How is it now?

Cole: Well in eighth grade I kinda got my act together. I wasn't living with Bettina anymore, I didn't see Caz or Bettina's daughters like at all. And I started talking to people and I started opening up, and I got, how do I say this, I started just trying to be more friendly and I wasn't a smart alec to people. I also liked my teachers a whole lot more and I could adapt to the environment a lot easier.

Elisabeth: Do you think that shift was specifically because you weren't living in a poly household anymore?

Cole: Yeah, I think a lot of it had to do with that. I think I just kinda got a life, uh more of a life. I had a lot of time to think and I had a lot of time to go out and meet more people, attend birthday parties, and you know just, I had a lot more fun. Eighth grade was probably, if it wasn't my best school year, it was either my best school year or this school year.

Elisabeth: Best how so?

Cole: I have friends now. And I can talk to people. And I get along with my teachers, I'm getting better grades. Let's see, I do better with my parents. But I'm still relatively well connected to the poly community. I don't know, part of it, I think a big part of it was her getting out and I think a big part of it was just getting my act together.

Cole had mixed feelings about polyamory—having to keep the secret or manage the information in such an enclosed social environment as a small private school clearly heightened his social awkwardness and made his tenuous relationships with peers even more problematic. At the same time, Cole felt that he had gained many personal advantages from his relationships with Bettina and Caz, and he valued his ongoing association with his local poly community. Perhaps most significantly, he acknowledged his own part in the difficulties, calling polyamory "the perfect scapegoat" for the consequences of his "smart alecy" behavior. In fact, throughout his interview, Cole struck me with his self-insight and willingness to own his part of a difficult situation. Characteristic of children in polyamorous families, he was articulate, reflective, and confident that his thoughts and ideas were important.

HOUSEHOLD CROWDING

In some families, children felt crowded and wanted more space. Zane Lupine remembered feeling crowded when growing up with his triadic poly family. "It was overwhelming sometimes, six people in a three-bedroom house. The adults shared a room, me and my brother shared a room, and my sister got her own room. Physically, I just wanted my own room and more privacy."

Zoe Hadaway felt a similar distress over a lack of privacy and had attempted to segment a portion of the large basement that housed the older children in the Hadaway family. Each adult couple had a large bedroom on the third floor, and the younger children shared rooms on the second floor, which left the large, semifinished basement for the older children—half for the girls and the other half for the boys. While her younger sister Michelle's bed was against the enclosed side of the staircase, Zoe had placed her bed in the corner and hung sheets, tapestries, and scarves as walls that delineated and screened the space from sight. Zany sighed, "Yeah, I think it is more fun for the little kids, to always have someone around to play with. But I am sick of always having everyone around, always having to share the bathroom, never having any privacy at all, even in the bathroom!"

Later, the family moved to a different house in the same neighborhood and redistributed the space. Several factors combined to allow Zoe to have her own bedroom, again in the basement, but this time:

> It has a door! I keep it shut most of the time. If I want to see people I go up and there they are. Otherwise, I'm in here and nobody can bother me. At least they're not supposed to. Before when I could never get any time alone it was a big problem. I could never have a private phone conversation, they were always wearing my clothes, going through my stuff. It sucked. Now they still try to go through my stuff but I'm going to put a lock on my door so they can't get in and take my stuff.

The negative effects of crowding appear to become increasingly acute as children age, and the teenagers seemed especially dismayed by their lack of privacy and space. For Jonathan Hadaway, it wasn't so much about privacy as lack of quiet. "It's really loud all the time with all of these kids," he said. "I can't sleep. They're all up too early."

FAMILY COMPLEXITY

For some people in polyamorous families the complexity of the relationships could be quite disadvantageous at times. These families experienced a number of complexities such as dealing with previous partners, jealousy and tension among siblings, difficulties adjusting to new parenting styles, adult drama, and difficulties managing information with families of origin.

Previous Partners

In monogamous relationships that end, people usually do not have to deal with someone close to them continuing to date someone with whom they have just ended a relationship. For Shelly and Sven Heartland, however, this was not the case. Initially they had formed a triad with Adam, but eventually:

> Adam and I [pause] broke up, I guess you could call it that, while he and Sven were still together. So he [Adam] and I were just friends

for the last like, two years of the relationship. It was a hard [break-up]. It was harder for me I'd say because I was really attached to him. And I just knew the whole dynamic was really going to change once it went from being a triad to just a vee. And it was hard, I mean, it was like any other breakup. Painful . . . He was primarily gay and had some bisexuality, enough that at the beginning it was OK. But as time went on he couldn't, he just didn't feel that way, you know, about me and all. And so we broke up and they [Adam and Sven] continued their relationship and we [Adam and Shelly] were just friends, and we adjusted OK. . . . It was hard because it was such a rejection, and then on the other hand I knew how much he cared about me, it was just on a different level, so, it was hard. And it was hard for him [Adam] too. I mean, we would both be crying when we were talking about it. I think he really wanted to make that part work too, but you can't make yourself feel something you don't really feel.

Elisabeth: Did it put a strain on your marriage?

Shelly: No.

Sven: No.

Elisabeth: How was it for you, Sven?

Sven: It is kind of probably what ended up leading to the breakup—my own breakup with Adam. It was stressful. I mean, we had good times, not that long ago we went on a Fourth of July ATV [all terrain vehicle, recreational riding] thing and it was fun, but it is just different. Because you start off being a triad and then you're not . . . The breakup [between Adam and me] started because it was not working with Shelly, and it just tumbled down from there, it kept getting worse and worse and worse until, attitudes . . . it was like a coin toss. He would come over and it was like, you never knew if he was going to be in a good mood and enjoyable or whether he was going to sit on the couch and be all pissy and grouchy.

Shelly: And everything changed. We went from him [Adam] coming and joining our family to them [Adam and Sven], it just being, if Sven did go down to [Adam's house], then he is away from everyone else.

While Adam's moodiness had been a factor previously when the triad was still together, it became more marked once he and Shelly broke up and there was more tension in the relationship. Going from a romantic to platonic relationship can be challenging for many people, but attempting to maintain a friendship when your ex-boyfriend is still dating your husband can be even more difficult.

Jealousy and Tension among Siblings

The intricacies of polyamorous families are complicated not only for adults but for the children in those families as well. Routine family challenges like jealousy among siblings can sometimes become even thornier when intensified by complex poly family dynamics. Zane Lupine reflected on his relationships with Pete and Joyce, his elder siblings:

> There is jealousy I guess, between my brother and sister and I. Because we have different dads, you know, there's always been that tension. Especially after their dad is not really that active in their life anymore, and my dad moved out here so he could be with us. There's just kinda always been a problem. But it's been a lot better, cause everyone's just kinda grown up and gotten over it.

Like many other families, children in poly families can have issues with their siblings, and these can be compounded by the effects of mixed parentage. In Zane's case, he shared the same mother (Melody) with his sister Joyce and his brother Pete, but Zane's father is Quentin and Pete and Joyce's father is Cristof. Mirroring experiences of other blended families with half- and step-siblings in serial monogamous families, the Lupine siblings felt some tension over the varying degrees of effort and number of resources each father was willing to contribute to the family.

Like Zane Lupine, Zoe Hadaway felt some friction with her siblings in her large, blended family. Prior to moving in together, before their parents formed the Hadaway family, Zoe and Michelle had been good friends. Combining households, however, took a toll on the girls' friendship. Zoe said:

We were best buds at the time and now we're sisters and so I don't know. Sort of like you can be best friends with somebody, then you move in together and you're like, that's a fault, that's a fault . . . We're still friends, but not like we used to be. Like it's like every single little thing we would tell each other before, and now it's just like you are really getting on my nerves and I am going to go shut my door in your face and you just have to go away.

In this instance, the parents' decision to move in together took precedence over their daughters' need for space to balance their friendship, which was strained by the intensity of interaction among siblings.

Adjusting to New Parenting Styles

Becoming accustomed to various parenting styles sometimes proved difficult for children in larger or blended poly families. Alvin, Jonathan, and Zoe Hadaway reported that their two fathers had quite distinct parenting styles.

Zoe: Yeah, both of the fathers are very dominant personalities. For kids who didn't grow up under them, when we were younger we believed almost everything we heard. We were very naive. Phil and Dad are, for the most part, the exact same person with completely polar opposite skills and personalities. They're both very smart alecy and they have quick reaction times. Mitch is mathematical and

Alvin: (interrupting) logical.

Zoe: Yeah, he's the logic stuff. Phil's very hands on, and Dad's [Mitch] not at all. He has no domestic talent whatsoever, besides that he's a very big leader. They fit easily into a leadership role. So the fact that I grew up in an academic-based household, where the head honcho [Mitch] was all business, "You make your money, do what you love, not because of the money but because you love it," and Phil was always, "We need to do this, don't question me. We just need to do it, we're going to fix it and make it work and . . .

Jonathan: There is no "because" from Phil, just do it. With Mitch there is a because, he explains . . .

Zoe: You could question him [Mitch] and he wouldn't be happy about it, but he would try to be logical with it.

Alvin: You could ask him questions, if you asked him a question he would answer it.

As the Hadaway children saw it, Phil and Mitch's clashing parenting styles wasn't the only source of conflict for the two men.

Adult Drama

In some polyamorous families, all of the extra communication and relational intensity translated to frequent arguments, and that was true for Mitch and Phil in the Hadaway quad.

Zoe: They just don't get along.

Jonathan: They have clashing personalities.

Alvin: Neither one would try to hurt the other; they just don't get along. I don't think it's as much of a problem between them, Jonathan is exaggerating, but . . .

Zoe: I would compare them to brothers, brothers that don't really get along. They get along sometimes, but they're always at each other's necks.

Alvin: It's back and forth all the time.

Jonathan: There's two alpha males living in the same household. Sharing a family.

Alvin: It's never like they're just helping each other, it's never like they are beating each other up either.

Elisabeth: Tension?

Alvin: Usually.

Elisabeth: Uncomfortable?

Alvin: Somewhat. But they kind of joke around with it, to make it seem more comfortable. They joke around when they are talking. The house, when the moms want to do something with it, he's like, "OK, if you think that's the right way to go, I'll be right with ya." If both moms agree then the dads will go along with them. Actually, it's usually the moms who have the final say for real.

Even with the joking around, there remained some family tension when the four adults would be fighting. Referring to her younger sibling Silas, Zoe reported that

he's finally reaching that age where he sees how hard the adult relationships can be on each other, and on the other adults. I remember crossing that line, where you finally start recognizing that the adults are really fighting. Even if you're not witness to the fights, you can tell when the adults are really not happy with each other.

Alvin: Dad won't sit with Mitch at cards, and the moms will do their things in silence. Tammy does her thing.

Zoe: Tammy is just completely quiet . . . she retires quickly. And when Mom's [Gwenyth] upset, she . . .

Alvin: the moms will get upset and . . .

Zoe: she tries to be as normal as possible.

Alvin: But then she melts down at other times.

Jonathan: It's there, that things are off.

Monogamous and blended families sometimes experience tension as well, though in this case the sheer number of people involved in a polyamorous family can create additional tension simply by volume of interactions.

Zane Lupine also reported that his parents argued regularly:

Zane: I guess the argument aspect could be a disadvantage. Cause there's more issues. More people, more issues. That's just how it goes.

Elisabeth: So did you have to deal with a lot of arguing when you were growing up?

Zane: Yeah, I'd say. Definitely not as much as some people do. I guess a decent amount. But whose parents don't, really, I guess.

Elisabeth: How did you handle it?

Zane: I used to think like, a lot of it was my fault, I'd worry about that. But of course they'd reassure me that it wasn't so eventually I just got fine with it. Of course it was a bummer, but it was never that big of a deal.

Elisabeth: So when it was happening what would you do?

Zane: Just go to my room and do my own thing. Just space it out.

Like many tweens and teens, Zane retreated to his private space to allow the adults to have their conflict unobserved. He distracted himself with music and homework or reading, and he left the adults to argue it out.

FAMILIES OF ORIGIN

Dealing with families of origin can present disadvantages to both adults and children. With four quite different sets of parents/grandparents, the Hadaway family had a wide range of families of origin with many differing beliefs. Gwenyth's mother, whom the children called Omi, lived in the area and became suspicious of her daughter's seemingly permanent "houseguests" as the couples grew closer. Eventually those suspicions boiled over into outright accusations after the two couples moved together to a larger home. Omi would see all of the grandchildren on what Jonathan called "a rotation, every weekend someone different goes to her house and gets to spend the weekend with her. There are nine kids, so a full rotation takes about two months to go through. But that's probably going to be on hiatus for a while, cause last weekend was so bad." When I asked what was so bad about last weekend, Zoe and Jonathan related the story of how Omi came to find out the quad was romantically involved. Zoe said:

> She was like, "I know what goes on over there and I think it's disgusting!" And I was like, "Well, that's your opinion!" and I stomped out of the room. But she would not drop it. It just got worse and worse. Finally she was like, "OK, we're going to dinner now. Come on, you said you wanted to go before." And I was like, "Actually I think I am just going to go home now." And she was like, "Don't do that." And I said, "I just want to go home now."

After a very awkward dinner in which "we didn't really eat much" and Omi "rambled on," trying to soothe Zoe's hurt feelings, Omi finally took Zoe home. Zoe reported that, on the way back to the Hadaway house:

> Eventually, Omi was like, "Don't tell your mom about this, OK? Don't tell her you're upset with me." Not that I had to. I walked in the door and mom said, "How was your trip?" and I said, "It was fine." And she said, "What's wrong?" I didn't say anything, I just came downstairs and put my bag away. By that time I finally broke down. Mom came down and said, "What happened" so I told her and it was bad. When I went back upstairs Omi was upstairs and Mom was still downstairs, and she [Omi] slipped out the door without another word. She knew that if Mom was down there talking to me, I was going to tell the truth.

> Jonathan: She [Omi] was like, "I need to go. She's [Gwenyth] going to be mad at me."

> Elisabeth: So when it happened the first time, she got information out of you? She kept pestering you?

> Jonathan: Like I said, she kind of has a way of just talking, she's getting information kind of without my knowing it.

> Elisabeth: What kind of information did you give her?

Jonathan: The thing is, she asked a question I didn't answer, which kind of told her it was a yes.

Elisabeth: What was the question?

Jonathan: "Do you think Mitch and Tammy have a relationship?" Actually, I think it was Zoe who she asked, "Why do Mitch and Tammy always sit in the front seats together?"

Zoe: Yeah, that was what she asked me. And then I came home and she asked me this. What was I supposed to do with that? Now she knows. It's like, "Jonathan, you have to go tell the parents. You have to let them know that she knows." Yeah. I was like, "You have to go tell her, Jonathan. If you don't tell her I will." And the way [the house was configured] with this great vaulted ceiling, the entire thing echoed . . . so whatever I said standing around in the doorway with Jonathan echoed upstairs and the parents heard it. They were like, "What's going on?" . . . So I went upstairs and it was like, "Omi knows. We need some damage control going on here."

The weight and intensity of keeping the family secret and managing older relatives' reactions to their unconventional family style was, in this case, emotionally painful and stressful for Zoe and Jonathan. Having to bear bad news and strategize about "damage control" can be burdensome for adults, and it is especially uncomfortable for children and young adults who have less control than their elders and may be unable to leave a difficult situation when they wish and end up having to sit through an awkward dinner.

In other cases, parents in polyamorous families fear negative consequences to their family complexity that never actually come to pass. When I first interviewed Shelly Heartland in 1999, she expressed concern that her daughter, Elise, might have to keep the secret about her mother's polyamorous relationship from her father, Shelly's ex-husband. Shelly said:

> What a terrible burden it could be if she [Elise] feels like she can't talk to her dad. He's kind of childish and unpredictable, he might be fine with it, or he might make a big deal out of it and use it to sue for custody. He was an ass during the divorce, wanted custody of Elise

just because he knew it would hurt me, and then didn't really even want to take her once he had gotten the legal right. Just because he was an ass to me and a mediocre dad most of the time doesn't mean that she shouldn't feel comfortable telling him the truth. So yeah, I worry that my poly relationships could make her have to keep secrets or other things like that that could be a pain in the neck for her. But we are concerned, because he is kind of volatile and I don't know how he would react with him, how he, knowing that she was a minor and we are seeing someone else.

When I interviewed Elise, Shelly, and Sven together in 2007, Elise dispelled the misconception that it was painful for her to hide her mother's poly relationships from her father. I asked Elise if she had any problem managing the information about her polyamorous family with "the school, with your friends, or your bio dad?," and she responded:

Well, he [Elise's biological father] really didn't know anything, really, the less he knows about my life the better. I lived out there for a year because things weren't going so well here and I thought I wanted to live in California. But let's just say I really, I guess it was a good eye-opener, but I don't think I would ever live with him again. So just the less he knows, the less questions he has, you know, he already has in mind what kind of a person I am and he's not going to change his mind about that . . . I think seriously if I tried to explain it to him he just wouldn't get it. Seriously, he's really naïve and closed-minded, and I seriously, when I go back there if we ever talk about anything I hear enough about the normal stuff he hates about you guys [Shelly and Sven], why add it to the fuel? He's just a bitter, hating man, very unhappy . . . When he found out I was moving back [to Shelly and Sven's place in another state] he flipped out. And at the airport, when he knew I was going back, he was like, he threw down my bags and was like "good luck" and left, that was it. He didn't even say I love you, nothing like that. So I don't know why I would say anything to him about Adam or my mom, why give him any more ammunition against us?

Rather than laboring to keep her mother's secret, Elise aligned herself with Shelly and Sven—"us"—against her father, whom she characterized as a "bitter, hating man." In this case, Shelly's fear of Elise having to keep her polyamorous relationships a secret becoming burdensome for Elise ended up being unfounded.

TOO MUCH SUPERVISION

Some, especially older, children from poly families expressed frustration at the degree of supervision they received from the numerous
adults in their lives. Not only did such surveillance hamper their plans
to sneak out at night or skip school but also children found that it was
extremely difficult to maintain a coherent lie when dealing with multiple parents. Marcus Amore found that multiple adults in the same
household made things more difficult when he attempted to lie to his
parents. While he felt that "I probably didn't even need to lie to them,
they were willing to allow me to do a lot of things as it was," Marcus lied
to his parents about walking to the local strip mall with his friends, but
without adult supervision. Marcus explained:

> When mom asked me what I did that afternoon I remembered to say
> that I got dropped off after practice and did my homework. Later,
> dad asked where I had gotten the [chewing] gum and I said I went to
> the grocery store with mom the other day and got some gum. Jim
> was sitting right there and said, "That's weird, I don't remember you
> coming with us." Mom, Dad, and Jim talked about it and could not
> remember when or where I would have gotten gum, so they asked
> me again and I tried to lie but it fell apart right away. They saw right
> through me, but I guess at eight or ten or whatever I was I was a
> pretty bad liar and having the three of them to cross check stories
> made it even worse. So it made it hard to lie, but it wasn't that big of
> a deal cause I hardly ever lied anyway, I just didn't need to.

Multiple adults providing supervision for children makes it more difficult for those children to do the kinds of things children do when adults
are not actively watching them.

Thinking back on her "rebellious phase," Elise Heartland reported:

> Sometimes it was a huge drag—I couldn't get away with *anything*. I
> mean, anything! The 'rents [her mother, father, and their partners]
> were always around, so if I tried to ditch school or pretend I went to
> practice [for the high school color guard] but went to hang out with
> my friends instead, someone would always find out. And if I tried to
> say I was somewhere else, somewhere I wasn't really, they would
> poke holes in my story. I would tell mom one thing and try to re-
> member what I had said to her when Adam (Elise's parents' boy-

friend) asked me how my day was, things like that. And they would talk to each other, so if I couldn't keep my story straight they would figure it out pretty quick. So yeah, that part sucked, but in other ways it was good to have so many people around, it kept me from getting into more trouble in high school.

Elise found the amount of adult attention she received to be both positive and negative for her. She liked it when there was always someone to pick her up or make her dinner, but she did not like the degree of supervision that kept her from "getting away with anything."

For Elise Heartland, too much supervision coincided with family complexity and produced an irritating level of adult intervention in her teenaged life. For Elise's father, Sven, he saw multiple adults in the household as an advantage because "Like if Shelly and I are arguing and I am being unreasonable about it, the third person can step in and say 'Sven, you are being unreasonable about this.'" Elise responded:

Elise: Yeah, but if you are a kid then you can sometimes have three people ganged up against you, telling you that, you know, you are being unreasonable, that really sucks.

Shelly: That's an advantage for us.

Elise: No, but if that extra person isn't your parent it really just pisses you off.

Shelly: I can see that, that is a valid.

Elise: (interrupting) I mean I used to fight with Adam a lot, like we used to, like "You don't have anything to say about that." But most of the time he was really nice and like really reasonable and I never had an issue with him, but if it was really serious about like us getting punished or something and then he would say something about it, it would just push me over the edge. It was like, "You don't even live here!" . . . Like when [Adam] would try to change from being a friend to like "I'm going to be on your parents' side now" and I would be like "What the hell?"

While Shelly and Sven saw Adam's additional interaction as helpful to their relationship with each other and their parenting, it proved to be disadvantageous for Elise when it translated to "three people ganged up against you."

In general, adults found the complexities of poly family life most difficult to deal with in terms of their increased vulnerability to authorities who might misunderstand their families and take their children away. Children also found family complexity challenging, especially when dealing with nosy relatives or peers at school who would not be misled with simple misdirection and continued to ask about the family. Like the other difficulties facing polyamorous families, these challenges are similar to the troubles that many families face, rather than being confined only to polyamorous families.

9

OVERCOMING OBSTACLES

People in polyamorous families use a variety of strategies for dealing with the disadvantages we discussed in chapter 8. These strategies focus on communication, emotional protection, stigma management, and being socially selective.

COMMUNICATION

Unsurprisingly, communication and honesty are chief among the practical polyamorists' tools for navigating their complex family lives. Poly families have frequent discussions, family meetings, smaller group chats, and one-on-one talks. If schedules are tight (as they often are), then the family meeting is a necessity because it can be otherwise virtually impossible to have everyone just wind up at home at the same time, awake, and able to focus on a serious conversation because they have no other pressing responsibilities in the moment. Many use the family calendar as a means of communication, because it specifies who is doing what and when and what people should expect from each other. Time carved out to be together routinely includes heartfelt discussions, and polys' first reaction to any issue is often to discuss it to see what family members think.

The Tree polyaffective triad consciously communicated about anything they could foresee as even potentially becoming problematic. In the hope that they could anticipate and defuse problems before they became bigger issues, the three would talk about their boundaries, feelings, and needs routinely. Such frequent discussion intentionally focused on dealing with issues when they were small and less charged, before they "blew up into big problems" as Leah put it, and this was a common strategy among polys. By being honest about their feelings and needs, addressing small irritations before they become larger, and communicating with each other frequently, the Trees and other polys use communication to check in frequently and keep everything moving smoothly in the relationship.

Shelly and Sven Heartland found communication useful when dealing with the departure of their beloved triad member Adam, whom the Heartland daughters Alice and Elise had come to adore. When Adam left and Alice was very sad, Shelly reported how the family dealt with it:

> We just kept talking to her [Alice] and saying, you know, we are not together in that same way and we still care about him and I am sure he still cares about us but he needed to make a life down there in [a larger town about sixty miles away] and he just can't really come up here any more. I just tried to explain as best we could.

Families used conversations to make sure the children felt that they could ask questions and express their feelings, so that the kids knew it was OK to miss someone. The pervasive expectation of honesty meant that children often felt comfortable asking their parents questions and expected a degree of candor that children in monogamous families might not have dared to ask.

EMOTIONAL PROTECTION

Parents' efforts to protect their children from the potential emotional pitfalls of polyamorous relationships took a number of forms, including carefully screening potential partners, training children in the realities of life, and prioritizing their relationships with their children above their romantic relationships. Poly people who are not parents also talked about using caution when dating parents, or simply not dating anyone with children if they are not prepared to establish a relationship with the child.

Screening Potential Partners

To counter the potential for their children to be hurt when partners leave, many poly parents use extreme caution when introducing new people to their children. In addition to taking the time to get to know potential partners through conversations, interactions, and observations, practiced polyamorists often check in to potential partners' relationship histories and ask other community members what they know of that person. Usually parents only meet potential or new partners outside of the home for extended periods of time until the parents are certain they can confidently introduce the new people to their children. Even once they meet the children, new partners are most often understood as friends and routinely blend in to the family's larger friendship network, especially at first. Usually the relationship only stands out to the children as significant beyond ordinary friendship if it lasts over a long period of time and reaches a level of significant or sustained intensity of emotion and interaction. In other words, polyamorists are not only quite selective about whom they date but also when and how they introduce people to their children.

Once they have introduced their partners, poly folks often encourage long-term partners to establish independent relationships with the children, relationships that occasionally outlast the sexual connections among the adults. Emmanuella Ruiz required her partners to establish a lifelong commitment to her children prior to being considered part of the family unit:

> I bring people into my life and there's a point at which I allow them the honor of being part of my family and I have great expectations from that and I expect the expectations of my children not to be dashed within that. So people are not allowed to come and go . . . I tell people if you get close to my kid, stay close to my kid. If you make a promise to my kid, it'd better be forever. So I'm very cautious about telling my children who is family and who is not. This person is mama's boyfriend and this person is family. So they know who they can trust . . . It's been going on for over a decade and it's working for all of them.

Emmanuella's caution and high expectations appeared to be effective in retaining emotional ties and ongoing supportive relationships among her extended chosen family.

Training in Real Life

Poly parents also talk about the importance of teaching their children
how to deal with the end of relationships as a valuable component of
emotional protection. Rather than make futile attempts to avoid loved
ones' departure, these parents seek to protect their children's emotional
well-being by teaching them how to deal with loss as an inevitable
feature of life. In discussing the impact of her divorce on her children,
Melody Lupine commented:

> It happens in everyone's life. The kids are learning that people come
> and go, but they're okay. And that it does not have to be this big
> thing . . . there's sadness but there's also joy when people come in or
> come back and that it can fluctuate, when people leave it does not
> mean forever.

Mark Coach similarly used communication as a tool to help his children deal with complex life issues, including those related to loss or
polyamory.

> I believe strongly that it is not a parent's job to protect their kids
> from the world. It is their job to prepare them for the world. To be
> effective adults in that world. Yes, that means you have to do what
> you can to insure basic survival and health. But preventing them
> from experiencing the pains life brings, that is robbing them of an
> opportunity to learn. It is much better to let them experience pain
> *and support them through it*. When I was fourteen my maternal
> grandmother died. My grandparents (from my point of view then)
> had been married since the beginning of time. They looked like they
> had the perfect loving, supportive relationship. (In retrospect I had
> no basis for making that kind of assessment, but I didn't know that
> then.) And yet, for all that perfection, she died, and he was left alone.
> That kind of loss, be it because of death or because of natural
> changes in relationship, is a part of life. I will have to deal with the
> loss of relationships. My children will have to deal with the loss of
> relationships. It is better to work through things, to support each
> other as a family, to experience loss and be supported through it, to
> learn how to ask for what they need, to learn how to share that pain
> with others who are being supportive, than to hide them from the
> pains they will have to deal with later.

Rather than what he felt certain would be a foolish and useless attempt at shielding his children from pain or change, Mark chose to communicate openly, to "experience the loss and be supported through it" as a way to help his children grow into "effective adults in the world." Poly parents express concern that attempting to insulate children from the inevitable loss of relationship that routinely accompanies life would actually be a disservice. Helping children develop the skills to manage loss or transition in many types of relationships, these parents hope, will provide more effective protection.

Prioritize Children

Poly parents routinely reported taking excruciating care to check out their partners, get to know people over time, meet people outside of the home, and prioritize the children in all things. Parents in the study discussed organizing their social lives and living spaces around their children. Logan Tex considered his eighteen-month-old son Pip and infant in every aspect of his relationships:

> Because I have my kids, I am more committed to Rhiannon [Logan's girlfriend] than I would be otherwise, because of Pip's relationship to her I am less likely to just walk away if things get hard. That being said, I wouldn't keep the relationship because of my son if things were really bad. It is a terrible mistake to stay in a bad relationship for the kids, baggage inherited from my dad.

Logan explained how children suffer in "bitter, awful homes" when their parents are in bad relationships that really should end but instead "hang on to the bitter end" so they can stay together for the children. It would be better to break up, Logan said, because "kids are sensitive to the moods of people around them, and if they grow up in an environment where people are always angry with each other, that would be damaging to them." For Logan and other poly parents (as well as many serial monogamists), consideration for their children looms large in their own relationship choices, whether that means choosing to stay with partner in part to sustain their relationships with children or choosing to leave partners who would negatively affect children either directly or indirectly.

If poly parents found that a relationship was having a negative impact on their child, they often ended the relationship. Claire Morgan, a
mother of one daughter, Renate, was firm in her conviction that Renate
was the most important relationship in her life: "It's a hard limit I have:
Nobody gets between me and my child." The extent of that limit was
tested, Claire reported, when her partner of over a year, May, began to
get increasingly irritable with Renate and became more controlling with
Claire, until:

> About three weeks before everything truly came crashing down
> around us, May and I went out to dinner, and she demanded that I
> give her full parental control over my daughter. She insisted that my
> health couldn't handle it [because I have a chronic illness] and that
> my daughter was out of control. That was one of those bucket-of-
> water-in-the-face moments, when you realize that someone is in a
> different reality than you are. Because, Renate, people love her . . .
> she's always gotten along well with people of all ages. People have
> pulled us aside to tell us how well behaved she is . . . But she and
> May were increasingly butting heads every time they turned around,
> and May demanded full control over Renate but there was no way in
> hell . . .

As Claire refused to punish Renate for misbehavior Claire thought
May had made up in order to manipulate the situation, May became
increasingly sullen until "she wouldn't even acknowledge Renate as a
human for over a week." That was the ultimate relationship violation for
Claire, who decided to leave as a result of May's mistreatment of Renate. Collaborating with her boyfriend Sylvester to "run interference"
and shield Renate from May, Claire immediately began to collect the
financial resources that would allow them to move out. May, however,
"beat me to it" and kicked the three out of the house they had been
helping to pay for but were not on the lease.

Claire was mystified by the whole experience, because she had been
quite careful when she established the relationship, and especially before she moved in with May. Claire said:

> This all happened despite the fact that we were very careful. I had
> known her for several years and we had spent more than a year very
> consciously working towards blending our households and making
> her a part of our family. Even so, we obviously didn't know enough

about her and didn't realize she had a narcissistic personality disorder. It wasn't until after we moved in together that things got increasingly strained . . . I still don't know what I could have done to avoid that. That could have happened in a monogamous relationship. I knew her in the community we shared, I'd known her for seven years before I moved in with her. There wasn't any kind of drama in our relationship. The only clue I had was that she talked a lot about an ex-partner who was supposedly stalking her. This person had left town, and I didn't know anyone who knew her or anything. Now I know, after doing some legal research, that she had basically done the same thing to another couple she lived with ten years before. She was arrested for domestic violence in that case, but she wasn't convicted so it wouldn't have come up even if I had done a criminal background check. Which I never thought I had to do. I do now, though, just to be sure. I'm very cautious, so much so that it kind of creeps me out. I don't like feeling this suspicious.

Similar to other poly parents, Claire normalized her relationship difficulties by equating them with the same kinds of difficulties monogamous families face and pointing out how poly families are better because they provide more resources—in this case, protection:

Like I said, it could have happened to people in a monogamous relationship too, I don't think it had anything to do with polyamory. Actually, having Sylvester helped us out a lot, he was something of a protection against May. I think she would have been worse and lot more likely to get more physical without him.

Considering the rarity of polyamorous families and the frequency of intimate partner violence (IPV), obviously most IPV happens between heterosexual, (ostensibly) monogamous people because they are the bulk of the population. While IPV is obviously a problem in some poly relationships, polys can use their contacts with multiple partners and social networks to ameliorate some of its impacts when it does happen. Because isolation is so often linked with one partner's ability to control another and perpetuate IPV,[1] people in poly relationships might be less likely to experience IPV because they are more connected to more people and thus potentially much harder to isolate. Multiple partners provide additional social resources that can help polys leave abusive relationships.

Claire's suggestion that Sylvester's presence kept May from escalating into violence deserves some additional consideration. It makes sense that people might hesitate to abuse their partners—something society has deemed deeply undesirable—in front of other people simply for the well-deserved shame of it. The presence of another person may not only embarrass the potential abuser but also may shift the balance of power if that person might be able to physically intervene on behalf of the partner who is being attacked. In case caution and slow negotiations fail to produce a reliably safe home environment, the strategies poly people use to deal with life events also have the potential to be benefits as well.

Nonparental Partners Caution

Poly parents were not the only ones who took great care with family interactions, and people who were partnered with parents routinely mentioned carefully monitoring or curtailing their relationships with poly parents in order to protect the children of those parents. After becoming close to Annabelle, Evelyn and Mark Coach's daughter, Kristine decided that she would no longer date parents:

> It's just too painful for me, for them [Evelyn and Mark], for the girls, especially Annabelle. I tried not to get too involved, but I just fell in love with Annabelle, she's a really special spirit. Then I tried to stay for her and for them, but that didn't work either for a variety of reasons. So now we're split and I hardly ever see Annabelle any more. When I do it's nice for me, I have no hard feelings towards Mark or Evelyn and I love to see Annabelle, but I can tell that they [Evelyn and Mark] are still tense around me so it is a little weird still. Yeah, I don't come over as much because of that, and because of that I have given up dating parents, at least for a while.

In order to protect her own and Annabelle's emotions, Kristine limited the time she spent with the Coach family, and she anticipated avoiding poly relationships with parents for the foreseeable future.

Like Kristine, Drew, a white man I spoke with at a poly potluck who appeared to be in his early to mid-twenties, told me he was not interested in dating people with children:

I'm too young for that. No one in my group has kids, so it's not that big of a deal, not like it's hard to avoid, but even if they were around I think I'd steer clear because I just don't even wanna start with that yet. Monogamous, poly, whatever, I'm just not ready to be that guy yet with anybody and it would just make dating so much more, uh, yaaaaaaa [claw hands] or something, like a whole nother person depends on this too. I'm just not ready for that at all. I'll definitely have kids later, but for now I really wanna, you know, check out what's out there.

In Drew's case, his youth meant he was not ready to take on an even quasi-parental role in any relationship, regardless of its level of sexual exclusivity.

Another way nonparent partners tried to protect the children in their lives was to attempt to foresee and avoid potential pitfalls. Some poly people were painfully aware of the potential for their attentions to the children of their partners to be misinterpreted and were hypervigilant in their attempts to make sure it was clear that they were not interacting sexually with the children. When Heather began to grow out of the small-child phase, James Majek reported that he was very careful to be excruciatingly appropriate with her:

> I see myself as a very important adult in her [Heather's] life and I'm very careful. For example, simple things like, we've talked very early on—Morgan, Clark, and I—it's been almost four years back now so Heather would have been six years old. I said I would not give her a bath, not because anything is going to happen, but because she might say the wrong thing to someone like "Oh yeah, that's James, he gave me a bath last night." Very, very careful; I will not give her a bath, and if I step out of the shower and she's around I'm putting on a towel because I don't want anything to screw this up.

James and other poly people in families with children—painfully aware of the vulnerable situation he and the Majeks occupied as polyamorous people with children—were extremely careful to prevent any misinterpretations of their interactions with the children. Aware that any misstep could "screw this up," James took special care to avoid even the appearance of impropriety.

STIGMA MANAGEMENT

Stigma threatens poly families from a variety of sources, among them adults' and children's peers; legal, medical, and educational institutions; and the parents of the children's friends. Poly people's strategies for stigma management include honesty, rejection of the stigma, normalizing the situation, and shifting stigma through education and patience.

Honesty

Logan Tex explicitly connected honesty and parenting with rejecting stigma: "Hiding our life would teach our kids that even close people are not what they seem, or that feeling shame for being who you are is appropriate somehow." By demonstrating self-acceptance and trustworthiness, Logan hoped to undermine the stigma associated with polyamory and provide his children with positive alternatives to counter any negative self-concept they might develop in reaction to conventional social expectations.

Honesty also reinforces the highly prized emotional intimacy between parents and children, an intimacy that parents use to shield their children from potential negative impacts of stigma. Many poly parents reason that, if they are consistently truthful, the children will trust them. Jonathan, a white father of three daughters in his mid-forties, believed that

> if I want them to deal in a forthright way with me, and everyone else in their lives, then I have got to demonstrate integrity by telling them the truth. It is an important thing, as a father, to be able to talk to them as much as they will talk to me. To let them be as much of who they are and love them for it, and show them who I am too.

For Jonathan, candid self-revelation is a marker of integrity, a way to establish trust with his beloved children, and the key to emotionally intimate relationships in which everyone was allowed to be (ideally) "as much of who they are" as possible. Rebuffing stigma, these parents offer their children an alternative view, based on a loving, authentic family with integrity. Families thus become havens of acceptance and sources of support, providing members with intimacy and positive role models to combat the harmful effects of stigma.

Rejection of Stigma

One of the most common strategies I found among poly families was the rejection of stigma, or refusing to identify with the perceived negative judgments of conventional society. Characteristic of this tendency, Tyler Warren—a white male high school student—refused to internalize negative social judgments about his family. When I asked him how things went when he interacted with peer's parents or other authority figures, Tyler replied that it generally went quite well, and that most of the time he had no need to navigate adults' negative assessments of his polyamorous family. Speaking of "regular people" who might negatively judge polyamory as immoral or somehow wrong, Tyler questioned the legitimacy of other people's judgments about his family, actions, or beliefs.

> You prove it to me how it's wrong. I'm doing fine, I don't need to prove anything to you, you're the one with the problem. If you have a problem with me or my family, show me exactly how it is wrong. It's up to you. Because I look around and I see love, I see caring, I see people living together pretty happily. Most of the time (laughing). What's wrong with that? If you have a problem with it, that shit's on you, not me. Innocent until proven guilty, isn't it?

Rather than taking on the shame he saw conventional society trying to project on him and his family, Tyler refused to absorb the stigma that others may "throw at me, screw them! Who are they to say? They lie all the time—like they can judge." Zane Lupine similarly rejected conventional society's judgments about his family:

> I've always been like, if they have a problem with that, that's their problem. I'm not going to hide it just so they can be comfortable. That's who we are. It's not something to hide really. It's fine with me. If it's not fine with them, then we shouldn't hang out.

In addition to defending his family from stigma, Zane used another common strategy I observed among youth in polyamorous families: normalizing the situation.

Normalizing the Situation

The majority of the time, life in poly families is boringly mundane, composed of homework, dinner dishes, and mowing the lawn. In such cases, it is not difficult to normalize the polyamorous family because the daily details of family life are normal in that they are the same things every other family does. Small children reflexively normalized the situation, meaning that their families seemed to them to be the de facto norm. True to their developmental stages, the young children between five and eight years old generally did not problematize their family forms but rather took them for granted as the norm. Older children were more likely to recognize the differences between their families and the more conventional families of their mainstream peers. For instance, Zane Lupine affirmed that his polyamorous family had been quite good for him.

> I think I've turned out fine, so I'd just use myself as an example of a successful relationship. Anything can go wrong in any relationship. Anything can go wrong in any raising of a child. If you have two persons in a relationship, that doesn't mean they're going to have a good childhood either. You can't guarantee it's going to be good for the kids, but you can't say it's going to be any worse.

In a way, Tyler and Zane's mutual rejection of stigma from conventional sources is simply age appropriate—it is a developmental hallmark of teenage years to question elders' assumptions and rebel against established norms. Both young men also grew up involved in poly communities, and their shared disdain for the judgment of conventional society was also influenced by their lifelong association with poly communities in which their families' style was celebrated and supported. Both spent large portions of their youth socializing with other poly families, where they did not have to hesitate or consider how to introduce their multiple parents. Their normalcy was taken for granted, and Zane and Tyler were able to compare their mundane poly family lives with the hellish tableau conservatives envision for multiple-partner families.[2] In normalizing their familial experiences, poly family members like Tyler and Zane engaged in what Pallotta-Chiarolli termed "polluting," in that they challenged the legitimacy of conventional or monogamous relationships "through noncompliance, personal agency, outing, resistance, and politicization by polluting the school world with one's bisexual and polyamorous existence."[3]

A very popular strategy among polyamorists wishing to reject stigma is to point out that the disadvantages associated with polyamory are not unique, and that monogamous relationships experience the same kinds of jealousies and complexities, only with the added layer of lying about it. In monogamous families parents argue, blended siblings crowd each other and have complex jealousies or rivalries, and people who used to be lovers struggle (sometimes unsuccessfully) to figure out how to co-parent. Most significantly, divorced parents involved in serial monogamous relationships have similar issues when people they are dating build relationships with their children and then leave. Logan Tex summarized a common poly response:

> We don't tell single parents OK, that's it, no more dating for you ever. But we do tell them to be careful, don't just invite people into your house and then kick them out again. But the model of denying yourself everything for the kid is not a good option either. Single parents, if they don't get to date to find a relationship, that is a sacrifice. Many humans look for a partnership with people, and to say that because you have kids you should not look for that or you will end up as a damaged parent. Because they can't celebrate their full selves, they are not going to be the best parent . . . the better place you are in personally, the better for you as a parent, and the better for the kid.

Logan not only normalized parents who date by pointing out the high number of single parents that society allows to date but also went a step beyond to imply that a fulfilled parent is superior to the self-denying, "damaged" parents who deny themselves romantic relationships and "can't celebrate their full selves."

While it is true that serial monogamous relationships experience disruption and single parents who date monogamously often break up with one partner and date another, what remains unclear is whether or not those things happen more often or more intensely with polyamorous relationships. Unfortunately, I am unable to answer that, and to date there are no statistics on the longevity of polyamorous relationships. As I have discussed throughout the book, my findings show both substantial romantic turnover (sexual relationships come and go) and significant relationship consistency (people remain connected outside of a sexual context) among poly folks.

Shifting Stigma

Some poly families were able to endure the stigma they faced calmly enough to educate the people who were stigmatizing them. For instance, Melody Lupine (Zane's mom) sought family counseling to deal with issues in her relationship with her then-husband Cristof. Initially the therapist was

> so judgmental. Oh, you know, "She [Melody] wants out of the relationship so she's getting involved with this other man and she's just prolonging it." And we're like, "No no no you don't understand. We're doing this thing called polyamory blah blah blah," and he's like, "Well, how about this other guy, is he willing to come in?" And we were like "Yeah, he's the one who suggested we come here." And he was like "What? OK, well, bring him in." He sat with all three of us and he was like, "Hmmm," he was baffled, literally scratching his head. "Well, bring in the kids" because he thought he would find pathology in the kids. So he interviewed the kids separately and then together and finally came back to the adults and he said, "You guys are on to something here and I want to learn everything I can about it." And he said, "If you work with me I'll work with you." And I thought that was huge of him and we, I ended up working with him for five years and he was such a wonderful man.

By reacting calmly and taking the time to teach their family counselor, Melody's family was able to navigate the initial stigma, neutralize it with education, and get the access to the counseling they needed. Their counselor gained a deeper understanding of polyamory and helped Melody to discover some profound personal revelations.

SURROUNDED BY SUPPORT

Many poly people are extremely selective about their friends and limit their social circles to those who will, if not actively approve of, at least accept their polyamorous families. In some of the families' social settings, their romantic configuration was irrelevant. Nonfriend classmates at school or colleagues at work, acquaintances, and random people the family members interact with in public settings do not need to know the details of poly family life and are routinely left to make sense of the poly family on their own. People with closer emotional and social ties are more likely to require (or be viewed as worthy of) an explanation, and poly family members tailor their interactions to the person and the setting. Deciding whom to tell and whom not to tell, people in poly families often blur their familial relationships with some people and explain them to varying degrees with others. In this section, we discuss the process of being socially selective in reference to stealth and secrecy, selective disclosure, and intentional socializing.

Stealth and Secrecy

Remaining closeted as a member of a poly family, or what some call passing,[4] was not difficult for the majority of the poly people I interviewed. Over and over I heard that, unless the person in question actively pointed out the fact that they were involved in a polyamorous family, others would simply make assumptions that explained the presence of various people in their lives and did not rely on polyamory to do so. As Adam Hadaway and Zina Campo's experiences illustrate, simply refusing to answer questions in some settings was all it took to derail peers' questions regarding family forms. In other cases, peers would not even know to ask questions because the poly family members would never appear at school, work, or other social settings that would possibly require explanation.

Dave Amore used a "don't ask, don't tell" policy with his former girlfriend Annabeth's parents, who would most likely not have approved of Dave's poly family or the quad Dave and Annabeth had previously established with their friends.

> Annabeth grew up in a Catholic family, though they're not necessarily practicing Catholics. She's not much of a person to believe in many religions, I think she's more agnostic than anything else. Her family had no idea about the quad, although I actually know her dad quite well and her stepmother. They don't know that I come from a poly family or that Annabeth and I have been in a poly relationship. It's never really come up in discussion; it's never been an issue. Which is

ironic, because I've been on several shows and Annabeth's actually told her parents about them. So, they probably "know" but they choose to ignore it. They've never discussed it with me, or with Annabeth as far as I know.

In this instance, it was not difficult for Dave and Annabeth to obscure the polyamorous nature of Dave's family, or Annabeth's relationship with Dave and the other quad members, even though Dave had appeared on several national television talk shows discussing his poly family. Annabeth's family tacitly agreed to ignore the things they did know and avoid asking questions or finding out any additional information.

Children in poly families intentionally seek out peers with whom they can safely be honest about their families. In many instances that meant peers who were adopted, had parents who were divorced, or had demonstrated their ability to be open-minded. Mina Amore said that she was honest about her family with her good friend, but not the friend's family:

> I guess I'm not necessarily what you would call normal, but who cares? Normal is boring. Some of my friends who seem really normal are actually super cool. My best friend, she's not normal either cause she's a Christian and her whole family really live like Christians, follow *all* of the rules that lots of people who call themselves Christian don't really follow. And we're Pagans, but she doesn't care. Her mom and Grandpa would *freak* if they knew about the whole Pagan poly thing—I mean *lose it*! But she doesn't care at all. We just do our own thing and are cool with each other. We're really different [from each other], but we don't care what other people think so we are kinda the same too.

For Mina and many other adolescents in poly families, normalcy appears to be overrated. Even things that may appear to be the norm, like Christianity, can become unconventional when practiced with fervor. The stigma that would otherwise accompany being outside of social norms does not necessarily translate as a disadvantage to those children (some tweens and many teens) who do not value conformity and who seek out peers with a similar disregard of convention.

Parents usually allow their children to use their own discretion when it comes to disclosing information about the poly family to the children's peers and other members of their social circles, at least to the greatest degree possible. Younger children who are possibly even unaware that they are members of poly families rarely have to consider issues related to disclosure, but elementary schoolers, tweens, and teens all have to make decisions about how to talk about their families to other people. Commenting on her children's social lives, Sara Bayside said:

> We let them take the lead, however they want to talk about it, they do. Their friends are pretty sophisticated, so I don't think it is generally a big issue for them. But we just keep our mouths shut about it, unless they [the Bayside daughters] ask us to say something, it just doesn't even generally come up that we're even in a position to deliver that kind of information to their friends. In general they run their own social lives, at seventeen and nineteen we are way past the play-date stage.

The Baysides' parenting strategy—allow their children as much freedom as possible within age-appropriate limits and provide backup when necessary—proved workable for them in many situations, poly related or not. That same strategy is popular among other poly parents as well, which is no surprise given the community emphasis on freedom and age-appropriate self-responsibility.

Intentional Socializing

Many poly families, especially those who live near large urban areas, intentionally socialize with other poly families to find friends and create community settings in which their families are unremarkable. As discussed in chapter 3, poly people intentionally seek community in order to get advice and support, look for partners, and find role models for themselves and their children who help to normalize poly families. Children told me they met other kids from poly families at poly campouts, movie nights, support group meetings, and dinner parties. By socializing with the same families over the years, these children are able to establish friendships with peers who do not judge their families and who immediately understand the relationships among the adults.

Even outside of poly social settings, children from poly families intentionally seek open-minded peers with whom they can become friends. Zina Campo reported that "I don't have to deal with it that much because I live out here on the farm with my dad, and mom and Blake live in [nearby town] most of the time, so it just doesn't come up most of the time." When I asked her if she had a hard time making friends while keeping the secret of her family's unconventional relationships, Zina responded: "Not really. Not at all. If they can't handle it I don't want to be their friend anyway." Zina and the majority of her peers in poly families seemed to easily control the flow of information with their peers and peers' parents, and Zina commented that "Only the cool ones get to know."

Zina devised a strategy that allowed her to talk about her friends from the poly community by saying, "Oh, those are just my mother's weird friends, they do whatever they want." Leaving the precise kind of weirdness vague worked well because "when I'm talking to my friends if an uncomfortable question ever comes up, that's one of the beauties of being twelve and thirteen, any bit of the conversation can just go away in like thirty seconds if you change the subject, so yeah, I don't have to deal with it hardly ever." This strategy allowed Zina to both maintain her privacy and respect her father's wishes for discretion with her "pool friends" from the local swim team that her father coached, as well a way to talk about the interesting things she did during the weekends she spent in town with her mother and their shared social network.

CONCLUSION

Implications for Serial Monogamy and Policies

Given the increasing diversity of families and the rising popularity of multiple-partner relationships,[1] as a society we must come to grips with a wider range of family formations and different sexual realities. Understanding polyamorous families provides us insight into how a range of families adapt to shifting social conditions. Some popular media pundits talk about poly families as if they are the sign of the death of civilization,[2] but they are mistaken. Rather than serving as the point of no return down the slippery slope of social decline to complete moral chaos, polyamorous families demonstrate an innovative flexibility that allows them to flourish in a complicated family style.[3] Society itself has become increasingly complex, with people living longer and more diverse lives—relationships must keep up with the changing social landscape. In this complex age, polyamorists have two very broad choices: 1) either learn the relationship skills, communication techniques, and at least a degree of self-awareness that it takes to have an ongoing poly relationship, or 2) leave the lifestyle. The learning process is ongoing, and the polys who choose option one are constantly doing just that—choosing and rechoosing, learning and practicing, never finished tinkering with ever finer points of relationship maintenance and emotional intimacy. Persistent polyamorists spend so much time working on, talking about, and perfecting their relationship expertise that they have

developed a range of useful skills that can be helpful to serial monogamists.

While poly relationships are not for everyone, their strategic innovations can be, because they offer insight into the unique ways people in
serial monogamous relationships can deal with their own blended families that mix multiple parents and children from past and current relationships. The tactics poly families have created, tested, refined, and
practiced can work for monogamous families who divorce, and their
experiences coparenting can illuminate how blended families of all
types might deal with multiple parents, regardless of how or if they are
sexually connected. This ability to adapt becomes increasingly important as divorce dilutes the expectation of permanent connections with
spouses and in-laws, while simultaneously creating multiple-parent
blended families.

STABILITY AND FLEXIBILITY

Families change. They have for the entire history of the human race,
and they continue to do so. Contemporary shifts in families are simply a
continuation (and acceleration) of endless variation, not the abrupt shift
from a previously homogenous and unchanging form of family that
some conservatives claim.[4] While the current prevalence of divorce and
single parenthood appear unprecedented, wars, accidents, and pesti-
lence have left many single parents across history.[5] Death used to end
marriages when life spans were shorter, and longer life spans means
more time for changes.[6] In an age when change is rapid and pervasive,
poly families are especially flexible and resilient, adept at surfing the
slippery and unpredictable currents of postmodern family life. Most
significantly, these families have developed ways to stay connected to
significant others among the fluidity, and they continue relationships
even as they shift form over time. By allowing their relationships to flex
with changing circumstances, polys are able to preserve ongoing links
with significant others and coparents.

Poly relationships may not last in the traditional sense of permanent-
ly staying in the same form. Instead, some poly relationships appear
more durable than many monogamous relationships because their flexibility allows them to meet shifting needs over time in a way that

monogamous relationships—with their abundant norms and requirements of sexual fidelity—find more challenging. While the familiar and
well-explored structure of monogamy can promote a comforting pre-
dictability, it can also limit the choices available to people in monogamous relationships. This is not to say that there are no relationship
innovators among monogamous people—feminists and others have a
long history of creating alternative definitions that provide meanings
outside of a patriarchal framework.[7] The scarcity of role models frees
people in polyamorous relationships to craft new relationships and in-
novate alternative roles that better suit their life circumstance in the
moment. Polyamorous relationships provide the flexible and plentiful
relationship choices that conventional monogamous relationships, with
their firmly defined roles and well-explored models, cannot.

Not only are poly families able to provide continuity across changing
circumstances, they also provide an ethical foundation to help guide
their actions. In other words, their fluidity does not mean they are
lacking a moral compass or that they are consequently adrift in a sea of
social chaos: These families have clear guidelines that prioritize honesty, compassion, freedom, and self-responsibility, forming an ethical
framework to guide interactions and decision making. These foundational ideas provide stability for children and adults. Unconventional
and frequently shifting, reliant on ethics rather than a conventional or
religious morality, poly families provide members with significant
stability while they flex to adapt to changing life circumstances. This
flexibility and willingness to explore alternatives makes some poly families uniquely resilient.

Family resilience researchers emphasize positive communication
skills and the cohesion of family network connections as key elements
that help families effectively weather crises. With multiple partners,
intricate schedules, and households that blend numerous parents and
children, polyamorous families face tremendous logistical and emotional complexities as they deal with the various challenges associated with
any family life, magnified both by the number of people involved and
the potential for discrimination based on their status as sexual minorities. Poly families' intentional expansion of familial roles and the self-
examination required by such deliberate innovation makes family members focus on cultivating the specific competencies required to navigate
complex familial circumstances and interactions. If resilience is "normal

development under difficult circumstances,"[8] then poly families provide a unique perspective on potentially difficult (or at minimum complex) circumstances. Strategies that allow families to adapt to changing circumstances are quite effective in contemporary society and would certainly prove useful to help more conventional blended families survive life in such a rapidly changing society.

Strategies for Monogamous Resilience

That is not to say that poly families are free of disadvantages—in fact they face the same disadvantages that other families face. Stigma, breakups, drama, teenage children who freak out, spouses who die—these are issues associated with contemporary family life. The advantages, however, significantly outweigh the disadvantages for most poly people who continue to engage in poly relationships. While the disadvantages are generally those associated with being in a blended family and occur culturewide, the advantages are specifically polyamorous. These advantages have helped long-term poly families to become uniquely resilient.

Poly people have established several strategies that can help people in families blended through serial monogamy to navigate multiple parentage and ongoing relationships with former partners. Divorce does not have to be so hellishly destructive, and if people are able to interact compassionately then they can have more resilient relationships that nurture positive coparenting even after they are no longer involved sexually.

POLY STRATEGIES FOR SUCCESS IN SERIAL-MONOGAMOUS RELATIONSHIPS

- Be honest early and often so you can trust each other. Communicate freely and frequently, and be honest with each other. Without those things, relationships will break down due to lack of trust, suspicion, and misunderstanding.
- Be willing to negotiate new ways to be; try alternatives. If the way things are going is not working for the relationship or family as a whole, be willing to consider doing things differently, and not just

differently from how you have usually done them, but differently even than most people do them. Be creative, and brainstorm a wide range of alternatives to make things better for family members and accommodate changing circumstances.

- Don't give up too soon. Put the best effort you can into making things work, and try your hardest. Don't give up, or as one respondent told me, "Don't mistake a bad situation or a rocky phase for a bad relationship." Consider alternatives you have not tried yet, and keep trying new things if what you are doing doesn't work. Find people you trust and ask for their support and advice. Get counseling. Give it your best effort, and assume the people who love you are trying everything they can think of to help things work out.

- Don't stay too long. If you have tried everything and the relationship still doesn't work in its current form, change it or end it before you hate each other. Do this before anyone lies to or cheats on each other, because it is much easier to trust someone and continue to coparent with them if they have not mistreated, lied to, or cheated on you, or if you have not done those things to them. It is important to change the relationship and end that phase in such a way that you can still trust each other and work together in the future.

- Redefine success. Monogamy no longer means what it used to mean. Even though most people who marry vow to be together "until death do we part," the popularity of divorce means that for many people that does not happen. These families do not have to be "broken homes"—outcomes for children and adults depend on how people handle themselves during and after a divorce much more so than the divorce itself. If you can successfully coparent and amicably attend family functions with ex and current lovers who are coparents, then that is success. Simply staying together is not necessarily success—it is the tone of the relationship that determines the degree of success, not just whether people remain in sexual contact with each other (or at least do not have sex with others) over the years. Success can be defined as meeting peoples' needs for a specific period of time. In such a rapidly shifting society, it is inevitable that things will change, and it does not mean people have failed. If people are able to accept change and handle transitions ethically, they will still be able to trust each other and coparent.

- Prioritize the children. Adults who become emotionally intimate with children should distinguish their parental relationships with their children from their romantic or emotional relationship with their coparent. All parents should consider and act on the basis of the children's best interest, and if the romantic relationship between the coparents changes or dissolves, then the coparents must prioritize their relationship with the child over any anger or desire for revenge they may feel. Ending a sexual phase of a relationship with a coparent does not mean that the relationship with the child must end or even suffer. In other words, adults' relationships to children should not depend on the adults' sexual interactions—adults can commit to cooperative coparenting without having a sexual relationship.
- Prepare children for the reality of postmodern family life. Many things in this society are in a constant state of flux, and learning to adjust to shifting circumstances is an important life skill. Be very slow and careful about introducing new people to children, do so in an age-appropriate manner, and clarify the status of the new person. (Is this person family or not? What should children expect from this person?) Let children know that people will come in and out of their lives—that is reality. Teaching children how to deal with inevitable fluidity is more effective than mourning the fact that relationships are impermanent. Help children to actively construct their own families, independent of adult whims. Provide them with the transportation, emotional, and financial support that enables them to see people that the children define as important—even if it makes the adults who used to have sexual relationships uncomfortable—so that children and young adults can establish lasting relationships with support structures outside of their parents' sexual interactions.

Underlying all of these strategies is the assumption that partners are negotiating as equals, which means women must have a framework that allows them access to economic independence, if not actual financial independence in the moment.

POLYAFFECTIVITY

Polyamory, the most flamboyant version of poly identity, is explicitly sexual in that it centers on being open to multiple sexual partners. A quieter version of poly identity, polyaffectivity appears to be more durable and flexible—able to supersede, coexist with, and outlast sexual interactions. Relationships that have such a multitude of options for interaction and define emotional intimacy as more significant than sexual intimacy allow poly people to craft a wide selection of possible outcomes. Most importantly, they allow polys to establish significant nonsexual relationships and maintain relationships over time even if their sexual content changes.

This expanded choice has two primary implications for poly relationships: graceful endings and extended connections between adults. Once a relationship can end without someone being at fault, the social mandate for couples to stay together and fixed in the same relational form at all costs can relax. As stigma subsides, the resulting decrease in shame and blame simultaneously diminishes the need for previous lovers to stay together until they have exhausted their patience and sympathy for each other, and possibly lied to or betrayed each other in the process. Once it becomes clear that the relationship no longer meets participants' needs or works for people who have grown apart, accepting the change and shifting to accommodate new realities can contribute to more graceful endings and transitions. If adults are able to amicably end one phase of their relationship, it increases the chances they will be able to make the transition to a new phase characterized by continued connection, communication, and cooperation. As one poly person stated, "Don't drag it out until the bitter end, disemboweling each other along the way. Split up while you can still be friends, *before* anybody does something horrible they will regret later."

A central component of polyaffectivity is removing sexuality as the hallmark of "real" intimacy. If sexuality can be shared among more than two people, and emotional intimacy can outlast or supersede sexual intimacy, then nonsexual relationships can take on the degree of importance usually reserved for sexual or mated relationships. That is, friends and chosen family members can be as *or more* important than a spouse or sexual mate. This extrasexual allegiance is fundamental to my concept of polyaffectivity and to the durability of these relationships that can flex and last over time.

Expanding important adult relationships beyond sexual confines, whether they be former sexual partners or polyaffective partners with whom there was never sexual interaction, provides people with more templates for interaction and choices in how to define relationships. One of the primary reasons to define the end of a relationship as failure is that it negatively impacts children. Bitter interactions among beloved adults are painful for children, and they aggravate the other emotional and financial disadvantages associated with divorce. Children don't care if their parents have sex, and they generally would rather not think about it at all. What matters to children is that they can have all of their parents at holiday and graduation dinners and that everyone is able to interact cordially. Ongoing positive interaction among adults is advantageous for the children in poly (and other) families because it means more support, harmonious family time, shared resources, and less money spent on lawyers.

This does not mean that no one in poly relationships gets hurt or mistreated in a breakup—poly people lie, betray, and cheat each other just like everyone else. But the existence of alternatives allows for relationships to end in one phase and begin in another, or continue across many versions that may or may not include sexuality. Expanding possible meanings, redefining success, deemphasizing continued parental sexual interaction, and focusing on cooperative coparenting provides options that can be advantageous for parents and children.

Allows Expanded Family

Polyaffectivity allows families to expand, and most significantly, it allows men more ways to be connected to families. Many families are in crisis; that is real. The predicament is worst for the children whose fathers act as merely sperm donors but provide little or no ongoing emotional, practical, or financial support. The crisis is among couples who attempt to sustain the weight of extremely high personal and social expectations on the narrow base of sexual attraction. It is abundantly clear that simple romantic attraction is inadequate to sustain a family over such long periods with life's complex and shifting circumstances. Expanding the base of family to a wider support, spread among more people who are connected by more than the potentially tenuous bonds of romantic affection, would provide a much more secure foundation for adults and children.

Spice

Multiple spouses need not be sexually connected, and indeed it appears as if the requirement that everyone involved must have sex with everyone else in the group (often accompanied by the expectation that everyone will love each other equally) can create unnecessary tension. The most lasting triads appeared to be women who were sexually connected with two men who were not themselves lovers but had significant positive regard for each other. Cowives or sister-wives have been common in many cultures across history and even recently on national television in the United States,[9] but cohusbands or brother-husbands are so rare that even the phrases themselves sound strange. Polyamory creates the opportunity for men to be spice in a way that they generally have not had access to in monogamy or polygamy, which is usually practiced as polygyny (one man with multiple wives) rather than polyandry (one woman with multiple husbands).[10]

Otherfathering

Just as revolutionary as allowing men to create emotional relationships outside of the stifling confines of traditional masculinity, otherfathering allows men to remain attached to children with whom they have developed emotional relationships. Although most of the people who bemoan "the crisis of the family" place it in the context of mothers who work for pay outside of the home rather than for free inside the home,[11] feminist scholars view it as a crisis of men in families who see true fatherhood as optional beyond sperm donation, as men sire children and then abandon them. Legislation pursuing "deadbeat dads" has attempted to make the men shoulder some of the financial responsibility for the children they fail to care for by garnishing wages and seizing tax returns. In the United States, we have taken a very punitive approach in our efforts to fix the problem of the absent dad, with much less focus on helping dads be better fathers. In other words, it is pretty clear that the stick approach has limited effectiveness, and I believe we should also try using the carrot as well. I am not saying we should repeal child-support enforcement legislation—on the contrary, we clearly need ways to make selfish or vengeful parents contribute to the children they create. But relying only on punishment and failing to encourage or recognize positive parenting and the attention of other loving adults who want to support children over time is lopsided and short-sighted. By recognizing and supporting the relationships men create with children, society can help them to sustain those connections over time and encourage men to remain connected to families and especially to children who love them.

Social changes have enlarged women's options and opportunities far more in the last sixty years than they have for men. Even though men remain firmly in control of finance, government, law enforcement, and industry in the United States and around the world, women have nonetheless made significant strides toward new opportunities and greatly expanded personal options since the 1950s. The same has not been true for men, and they remain almost as bound by the expectations of traditional masculinity as they were sixty years ago. Not only have their clothes barely changed, but their personal, emotional, and expressive options have not expanded on par with women's. This is due in part to women catching up with the options that men already had, and in part to the rigor mortis that seems to have set in around conventional masculinity. As a society we give lip service to approving of stay-at-home dads and men who are able to cry, but it is a grudging and shallow approval that stops well short of actually valuing gentle, empathetic, and kind men. Contemporary ideals of masculinity in the United States remain firmly rooted in aggression, and it is the chiseled features of the muscular hero able to escape the building moments before it detonates that capture our imaginations, not the devotion of a man to his children against all odds. Movies about relationships are still chick flicks, and movies about men are really about action—as long as something explodes they are in tediously familiar territory.

The problem is that this familiar territory is stifling and cramped, far too limited to accommodate the true range of men that exist and the choices they make. While laws focus on punishing men for their (admittedly grievous) failings and popular culture celebrates a very limited, pale, and muscular version of masculinity, poly men and people like them are quietly expanding the boundaries of what it means to be a man in a family today. Allowing women into positions previously reserved for men has expanded their choices, but it has not made positions traditionally held by women (like those associated with caring for a family, including the cooking and cleaning) become more valuable. As a society we take it for granted that women will care for their children, and we are still amazed and overjoyed when men change a diaper.

Many men in poly families take *real responsibility* for their children and continue to nurture supportive relationships with children—even once they no longer have sex with the children's mother. That is precisely what society has expected from women all along—that women prioritize their relationships with their children over their sexual relationships with men. Women who fail to do this are severely stigmatized and are branded whores and bad mothers. Applying that same standard to men is revolutionary and worthy of social and legal attention, because these men establish relationships with their children (even children with whom they do not share a genetic link) independent of ongoing sexual relationships with their mothers.

Expanding men's social and legal options can help them stay connected to families and supporting families in general by valuing the functions and parts of family usually viewed as women's work. The more men do what previously was women's work, the more valued it will be. If the real responsibilities of caring for children continue to fall only to women, then too many children will remain in poverty and emotional need. It is only when men are also as deeply responsible for children as are women that the kids will have the benefits of a wide base of support. It would be better for children, and for the many men who are unable or unwilling to live up to the requirements of conventional masculinity, if we could allow men's personal, emotional, and relationship choices to expand as much as we have allowed women's to increase.

POLICY IMPLICATIONS

On the most basic level, public policies should help the people who live in the society that the policies regulate. That means assisting the people who actually exist, rather than bemoaning the fact that they are not the people who used to exist or lawmakers might prefer to exist. At minimum, policies should not hurt families or hinder their attempts to cope with crises. Extending the same marriage benefits to people in same-sex and polyamorous families (and others) as those available to people in heterosexual couples would be a good start in supporting contemporary families. Even though many polyamorists and some lesbians and gays scorn multiple or same-sex marriage, in the interest of full citizenship and equality they still deserve to have the opportunity if they decide they want to marry. Encoding second-class citizenship into marital laws only further alienates already disenfranchised sexual minorities and perpetuates institutionalized homophobia. Worse yet, it hurts the children from those families.

Rather than evidence of decline, polyamorous families are a symptom of a society that is constantly and rapidly changing. It is clear that the singular family model of the monogamous, heterosexual couple linked by romance alone, precariously perched on their unwavering emotional, sexual, and financial investment in each other, does not work for everyone. As numerous divorce studies illustrate, for at the least 40 percent to 50 percent of all marriages that experience a "disruption,"[12] one size no longer fits all, and blended, serial monogamous, same-sex, and polyamorous families are here to stay. Policies and laws should catch up to serve society as it actually is, rather than punishing people who do not fit the white, middle-class, heterosexual, monogamous model of sixty-five years ago. For some people, family forms with broader foundations are more flexible and resilient, better able to meet the complex needs of diverse contemporary lives. It is wiser for some, especially sexual minorities, to invest their long-term emotional and financial care and parenting arrangements in relationships with friends, siblings, or platonic coparents.[13] Policies and laws should legally recognize and serve these families.

Are same-sex or polyamorous marriages truly so terrifyingly powerful that their mere presence could obliterate heterosexual, monogamous marriage? I think not. Marriage based on monogamous, heterosexual couples is and will probably continue to be a very popular form of relationship in some regions of the world. Because the majority of the population is heterosexual,[14] it is clearly better suited to more people than same-sex marriage. Monogamous marriages can also be less complex, offer more plentiful conventional role models, and earn greater social approval, making them more appealing for many people than the potentially more complex and high-maintenance polyamorous family.[15]

Policy Recommendations

One thing this research makes abundantly clear is that our social and institutional framework can no longer shape itself to serve the legally married heterosexual couple with nondisabled children, a dad who earns enough to support the entire family, and a mom who "doesn't work" (meaning she provides free home and child care). Certainly some people marry and maintain one paid worker and one stay-at-home parent who (at least for a time) leaves the paid workforce in order to take care of the children, but these families are no longer the majority. Families with a full-time earner and a full-time parent are the statistical minority, but current policies are still designed to serve families as if everyone with children has a full-time caretaker at home. Shifting policies to better serve families as they are, rather than how we imagine them to have been decades ago, will not undermine heterosexual, dyadic families—they will still be covered under health insurance policies, inheritance laws, and hospital regulations.

Refocusing laws, regulations, and policies on children, rather than the adults to whom they are related, would far better serve the diverse families that actually live in the United States today. If a child is in poverty, lacks health care, clothes, or food, that child should get assistance regardless of the status of the child's parents. Rather than concerning themselves with who lives in the home or if the child's mother has a marital/sexual/any relationship with the child's father, policies should be based on what is best for the child. The monogamous heterosexual family is no longer the sole family form, and policies need to evolve beyond partisan squabbling about religion and sexuality to providing for children who will be the future of our society, regardless of their parents' sexual relationships or lack thereof.

In addition to focusing policies and laws on children's needs, this research highlights a need to shift laws regulating child custody and adults' relationships. Currently, there can be only two legal parents of any child, and if someone else seeks to become a parent, then one of the other parents must relinquish parental rights prior to the new parent being legally recognized.[16] Rather than making it more difficult for adults to attach to children, policies should allow multiple adults to be legal parents to the same child in order to distribute the extensive emotional, practical, and financial needs associated with raising a child among multiple adults. By officially recognizing multiple parents, policies can help to attach more adults more securely to children. As this research has repeatedly demonstrated, pooling resources allows families to meet a wide variety of children's and adults' needs, and far too often children's needs go unmet.

Obviously, multiple parents can introduce additional complexities, which would require courts and policymakers to create new ways to manage the complexity. I suggest assigning parents to specific portions of the child's life that best fit the specific parent's strengths: educators should be in charge of the children's education, medical professionals should be the chief decision makers when it comes to medical issues, and the primary caretaking parent should have the most say in disciplinary situations. With rights come responsibilities, and these additional parents would be responsible for supporting the children financially as well as emotionally and physically.

Second, policies should expand to recognize multiple levels of relationships among adults. Currently, most laws and regulations recognize a very limited range of relationships—primarily biological relatives or legally married couples. To more effectively support contemporary families, laws should recognize connections between and among significant others like siblings, cohusbands, or lifelong friends who function as family members. By recognizing adults' relationships, laws can support connections between and among adults who are attempting to care for children or each other. In a society with a crumbling social safety net, the more ways in which people can care for each other the better. Polyamorous families provide examples and innovations that can help serial-monogamous families navigate postmodern family life, and as a society we should attend to their innovative ideas that can prove useful for other families as well.

APPENDIX A

List of Recurring Families

Amore: Louise, Max, and Valentino; sons Dave and Marcus, daughter Mina; Louise's mother JP

Ballard: Geoff, Hillary, and Jake; daughter Marni, son Milo

Bayside: Calbair, John, and Sara; two grown daughters**

Bien: Warren, Andrew,** Devon,** Estella,** Julie;** daughters Rebecca,** Callie,** and Macy**

Campo: Samuel, Blake, and Lexi; daughter Zina; Lexi's mother Dia and father Brian

Coach: Evelyn, Kristine, Mark, Marshall, and Regan; daughters Annabelle and Martine**

Cypress: Howard and Josephine; son Cole

Founder: Jana, George,* Michelle,* Mike,* and Sam;** son Zachariah*

Hadaway: Gwenyth, Mitch, Phil, and Tammy; ten children including
Daughters: Amelinda; Bunny, Candace, Lily, Michelle, and Zoe
Sons: Adam, Jonathan, Nick, Silas

Heartland: Adam, Richie,** Shelly, and Sven; Daughters Alice, Elise, and Kimber*

Holstrom: Billy, Jack,* Megan,* Sabine,* and Tad;** daughter
                Ariel,* sons Nolan* and Simon**

Kenmore: Dax, Iris, Natalie, and William; son Dillon

Lupine: Cristof,* Melody, and Quentin;* daughter Joyce, sons
              Pete* and Zane

Majek: Clark, James, Morgan, and Nash; daughter Heather,
             sons Brady,* Beck,** and Sebastian

Mayfield: Alicia, Ben,* Monique, and Edward; daughters Josie and
                Kate*

Omni: Baldwin and Nadia;** daughter Rosaline,** son Wade**

Phoenix: Jared, Summer, and Zack

Rivers: Rebecca; daughters Clarabelle and Eliz

Ruiz: Emmanuella; three grown children

Starr: Joya; son Gideon*

Taylor: Ada and Jasper; daughter Octavia and son Xander

Tex: Logan, Melina,** and Rhiannon;** two children, Pip (17
           mos) and infant**

Tree: Bjorn, Gene, and Leah; son Will**

Warren: Dani, Lex, and Mike; son Tyler

Wyss: Albert, Kiyowara, Loretta, Lucia, Patrick, and Fred;
            daughter Kethry, son Evan*

*Denotes a family member with participant observational data but no
interview.

**Denotes a family member with no interview or participant observa-
tional data.

Please note that any respondent whose name is bolded and appears at
the beginning of the listing, out of alphabetical order, is the sole respondent from that family. In such cases, I list the respondent first to be
clear that they are constructing their entire data line, and other family
members did not participate. Most of the time I was able to interview

and/or observe multiple members of the same family, and in those cases their names appear in alphabetical order.

APPENDIX B

Research Methods

While I will be using more academic language in this section, I encourage everyone to read it even if they are not academicians. Please do not be afraid of the language—these are simply words that describe ideas, and readers are capable of grasping these concepts if they allow themselves a bit of time and patience with themselves. Thinking critically about research results presented as "facts" in news media, radio talk shows, and online discussions means being able to put that research in context to understand its potential strengths and weaknesses. Critical thinking also means a more informed, thoughtful, and meaningful public dialogue—something we are clearly lacking in large sections of our cultural sphere. In this book, I have made every opportunity to put the respondents and myself in social context so readers can think critically about the research findings. What follows are more details about the research methods I used in the Polyamorous Family Study.

THE STUDY

This book is based on a fifteen-year qualitative, ethnographic study of people in polyamorous relationships that came to focus increasingly on families with children. I collected the data in three waves using several different research methods. A very common strategy among ethnographic researchers, I began with *participant observation*—basically hanging out with poly people, chatting with them, and watching how they interact with each other in their "native" social settings of public meetings, support groups, "meet-ups" in local restaurants, group hikes, movie nights, and "potluck" dinner parties hosted in private homes. I also used *content analysis*, in which I documented common themes in the poly people's books, magazines, and blogs that I read. Using the Internet allowed me to *read discussions and interact with people on poly list-serves*. One specific list-serve, Polyfamilies, was already focused on what I was studying, and it proved quite responsive to my questions. Routine interaction with that list-serve evolved into a kind of ongoing, slow-motion focus group with some people participating a lot, others commenting occasionally, and many simply following the discussion or "lurking." Some of those conversations are documented in this book, always with the original author's permission. Finally, I used in-depth *interviews* that began with routine questions about how the person defined polyamory, how they initially got involved, and their past and current relationships. From there, each interview followed whatever the interviewee felt was most important to discuss. People who participated in the second two waves of data collection also filled out demographic *questionnaires* that asked questions about their age, race, sexual orientation, occupation, (dis)abilities, and gender identity.

Three Waves of Data Collection

Wave one (1996–2003), my dissertation research, included participant observation with roughly three hundred people and forty in-depth interviews (twenty women, twenty men) with adults who identified as poly, with one sample in the Midwest and another in the California Bay Area. During this phase I attended a wide variety of poly events, especially frequenting a monthly poly women's support group and attending two national conferences sponsored by the Loving More organization. In what turned out later to have a significant impact on the follow-up study, the Institutional Research Board (IRB, a committee at every research university in the United States that oversees a professor's research to make sure it is safe for the people who volunteer to participate) at the University of Colorado decided that the interviewees would be safer from being accidentally exposed as sexual minorities if I did not keep any identifying information on them. The only records the IRB allowed me to keep from the original study were the pseudonyms the interviewees had chosen.

The second wave of data collection (2007–2009) did not begin until four years later, in part because the IRB at Georgia State University discussed it in many of their committee meetings and they required frequent (sometimes opposing) revisions to the research protocol (a document that describes the methods I planned to use and how I would protect respondents' identities) before they would allow me to begin the research again, keeping contact information this time. The greatest obstacle to continuing my research was the IRB's reluctance to allow me to talk to children, so I deleted that component of the research plan and was finally able to meet their requirements.

Once I got IRB approval, I posted messages on as many of the poly websites and list-serves that would allow me, asking people who had participated in the first wave of research to email me so I could follow-up with them. This initial Internet call resulted in seventeen previous respondents emailing me, with fifteen of them consenting to interviews. I also interviewed their partners and one adult child, expanding the sample to include an additional thirty-one adults. Interviews in this phase focused more on managing family life and interacting with social institutions such as schools, medical establishments, and child welfare agencies.

The fact that less than half of the first sample responded again in the follow-up study means that the perspective of those people who did not participate is missing from the research. Because I used poly community connections to look for people (the only way I could think of that was realistically within my budget and allowable under university research guidelines), and the people most likely to stay connected to the poly community are those who still live a poly lifestyle, this research emphasized continued involvement in poly families and community relationships. It is highly likely that some of those people who did not participate dropped out of the poly community because their poly relationships did not work out. With the exception of Melody Lupine, their perspectives are missing from the data.

While I was collecting the second wave of data, I was also revising my research protocol and meeting with the IRB officials at Georgia State University in an effort to get their permission to talk to children—

a feat that took three grueling years and resulted in research protective practices that one IRB committee member privately confided he thought were "ludicrous and paranoid." As past academic abuses indicate, it is important to protect people who participate in research, and IRBs across the nation serve a valuable purpose. In this case, however, sex negativity (fear of and disdain for sexuality or anything related to it) clouded the Board's judgment, made the process far more difficult and time-consuming than it needed to be, and significantly hampered my research process and output.

As soon as I received permission to interview children, I began the third wave of data collection (2010–2012), which included twenty-two children and thirty-eight new adults, as well as former respondents participating in follow-up interviews. The third wave focused primarily on children and their important adults, and interviews continued on the same themes of family life and interactions with social institutions. I also relied more heavily on participant observation in the third wave of the study, watching small children too young to participate in interviews and observing family interactions between kids and adults, and among children.

Data Analysis

In quantitative research, data usually comes in the form of numbers, and findings often appear as percentages. Qualitative research (such as this study) produces data in the form of words, and the researcher's goal is to find trends and patterns in what the people said, where they contradicted each other, and the many different ways in which they experience or understand their lives. To analyze the data from this study, I used a modified form of grounded theory that began with *inductive data-gathering* methods, where the questions I asked grew out of the environment I studied (rather than deductive research that begins with a hypothesis and then checks to see if it is true). Once I got started, I used *constant comparative methods* to analyze the interview data and my field notes with a process that included (1) reading transcripts and generating initial coding categories (broad categories such as *interaction with peers* or *experiences of jealousy*), (2) identifying and relating similar ideas and the relationships between and among categories, (3) adjusting these analytical categories to fit emergent theoretical concepts, (4) collecting additional data to verify and/or challenge the validity of those concepts, and (5) probing these data for the boundaries and variations of common themes. This process allowed me to constantly refine my questions and understand the nuances of complex ideas that I had first begun to grasp in the early portions of the research.

While many researchers use the methods described above, I added my own twist by sending drafts of what I wrote to respondents so they could see how I was using their words. This gave them an opportunity to correct anything I had gotten wrong (which happened only rarely and tended to concern details such as whose birthday it was or whose parent said what), to update information, and to include additional thoughts. This combination of constant comparative methods and a feminist research framework that empowers respondents to actively participate in and shape the research process was available to me only because email allowed such easy communication and document sharing.

The Sample

The total sample for the study is 131 interviewees and five hundred participants observed. Some respondents I interviewed or interacted with only once, and others I interviewed up to four times and interacted with over fifteen years. Race was the most homogeneous demographic characteristic, with 89 percent of the sample identifying as white. Socioeconomic status was high among these respondents, with 74 percent in professional jobs. Fully 88 percent reported some college, with 67 percent attaining bachelor's degrees and 21 percent completing graduate degrees.

Defining polyamorous families is challenging, not only because social scientists and members of the public disagree on the definition of families but also because poly community members dispute the precise boundaries of what it means to be polyamorous. For this study, I included people who self-identified as polyamorous, and in this book I focus on those who identify as members of poly families. There are many respondents without children or connections to families with children who do not appear in this portion of the research, but they are more evident in some of my earlier publications on polyamorous women (2005) and polyamorous men (2006).

Names

As with most research, I used *pseudonyms* (fake names) for people in the study to help protect their identities. Many of the participants selected their own first names, though I eventually changed some of the most unusual ones to more conventional names when several different editors mentioned that the eccentric names were becoming a distraction from the content of what the people were saying. As the book evolved, it became clear that keeping track of all of the different people in each family was becoming increasingly confusing, so I made up last names for each family group. In reality, all family members very rarely share the same last name.

A FINAL NOTE TO READERS AND RESPONDENTS

While I made every attempt to explain these families in as great a detail as possible, it is very difficult to squeeze fifteen years of research into a single book. Of necessity, most of what people told me has been left out. In order to give the respondents an opportunity to add important information and possibly tell an entirely different side of the story that does not appear here, I am collaborating with the Woodhull Sexual Freedom Alliance on the Family Matters project. Woodhull has offered a special section of the Family Matters website for respondents of the Polyamorous Family Study, which you can find at http:// www.familymattersproject.org/. If you participated in the research and would like to elaborate on something in the book or provide a different perspective, please email me at dr.elisabeth.sheff@gmail.com and I will give you instructions on how to access that part of the site. If you are a reader who wants to follow the people in the book, please visit the *Polyamorists Next Door* section of the Family Matters website, and consider posting about your own family while you are there.

NOTES

INTRODUCTION

1. Please see Appendix B for a more complete discussion of the research methods I used for this study.

2. I would always ask these people if I could quote them, either in person if we were chatting or by private email if I was quoting them from an online discussion.

3. *Loving More*, http://www.lovemore.com/magazine/.

4. (Popenoe 1996; Waite and Gallagher 2000; Wilson 2002)

5. (Coontz 1988, 1992, 1998, 2005; Skolnik 1991; Stacey 1996)

6. (Coontz 1992, 1998, 2005; Skolnik 1991; Stacey 1996)

7. (Baxter et al. 2005)

8. (Amato 2001; Hetherington & Stanley-Hagan 1999)

9. (Bumpass & Raley 1995; Edin & Kefalas 2005)

10. (Carrington 1999; Stacey 1996, 2003)

11. (Sullivan 2004)

12. (Bartell 1970, 1971; Fang 1976; Henshel 1973)

13. (Denfeld and Gordon 1970; Spanier and Cole 1975)

14. (Constantine and Constantine 1973; Smith and Smith 1974)

15. (Rubin 2001)

16. (Anapol 1997; Anderlini-D'Onofrio 2005; Block 2008; Easton & Liszt 1997; Nearing 1992)

17. (Sheff 2011)

18. (Sheff 2011)

19. (Rubin 2001)

20. (Bettinger 2005: 106)

21. (Riggs 2010)
22. (Pallotta-Chiarolli and Lubowitz 2003)
23. (Pallotta-Chiarolli 2006)
24. (Pallotta-Chiarolli 2010a)
25. (Pallotta-Chiarolli 2010b)
26. While ideally people in serial monogamous relationships break up with one person before beginning a new relationship with someone else, in practice many people actually establish another relationship prior to breaking up with their current partner.
27. (Olsson et al. 2003)
28. (McCubbin & McCubbin 1988)
29. (Olsson et al. 2003; Patterson 2002)
30. (Patterson 2002: 240)
31. See http://www.kerista.com/ for more information on Kerista.
32. http://www.kerista.com/
33. http://en.wikipedia.org/wiki/Morning_Glory_Zell-Ravenheart
34. http://en.wikipedia.org/wiki/Oberon_Zell-Ravenheart

I. WHAT IS POLYAMORY?

1. For more discussion on the importance of gender in polyamory see Ritchie and Barker 2006; Sheff 2005a, 2005b, and 2006).
2. (Aviram 2007)
3. See Sheff and Hammers, "The Privilege of Perversities," in *Psychology & Sexuality* 2, no. 3 (2011) for a more comprehensive discussion of the racial and ethnic composition of polys in the United States, Europe, and Australia.
4. Tantra is a form of sacred sexuality originally associated with a form of medieval Buddhism in India, introduced to the West in the 1960s and popularized in a much-Westernized form in Australia, Canada, Europe, and the United States.
5. Ages were current at the time of the interview, not the time when the people met.
6. Although my data includes information regarding two separate moresomes of twenty gay men in each, gay men are rare in the communities I studied, and moresomes this large are even rarer, especially ones that own large houses together. The appearance of two moresomes of gay men who own homes together is anachronistic in the polyamorous communities I studied. My sample is not representative of men who have sex with men. For more detailed information on that population, please see Yip (1997), Connell (2005), and Weeks, Heaphy, and Donovan (2001).

7. http://aphroweb.net/articles/nre.htm

8. Ken Haslam is a well-known polyamorous activist who speaks publicly and sponsored the polyamory collection at the Kinsey Library at the University of Indiana, http://www.kinseyinstitute.org/library/haslam.html.

2. WHO DOES POLYAMORY, AND WHY?

1. (Sheff and Hammers 2011)

2. Polyamorists in the United States have adapted these forms of sacred sexuality; neither traditional Taoism nor Tantra advocate multiple-partner sexuality. There is no traditional form of Quodoshka; it is an amalgamation of several different Native American traditions created in the late twentieth century, practiced primarily by middle-class, white "new agers." Many polyamorists critique Quodoshka as heterocentric and monocentric; still, some have adopted it and seek to adapt it to polyamorous relationships.

3. http://www.poly-nyc.com/

4. http://www.kinseyinstitute.org/library/haslam.html

5. V. Foster, P. C. Clark, M. M. Holsad, and E. O. Burgess, "Factors Associated with Risky Sexual Behaviors in Older Adults," *Journal of the Association of Nurses in AIDS Care* 23, no. 6 (2012): 487–99. doi:10.1016/j.jana.2011.12.008

6. Nancy Levine and Joan Silk, "Why Polyandry Fails: Sources of Instability in Polyandrous Marriages," *Current Anthropology* 38, no. 3 (1997): 375–98.

7. (Sheff 2005a)

8. (Connell 2005)

9. (Sheff 2006)

10. (Ritchie and Barker, 2006)

11. (Collins 2000)

12. In this work I primarily use the term *African American* when referring to people of African descent, though when the respondents use *black* I do as well in order to mirror their language.

13. For a more detailed discussion of the role of race/ethnicity, social class, and education, as well as the impact of research methods on sexuality research, see Sheff and Hammers 2011.

14. (Gould 2000)

15. I took scrupulous care to use neutral wording when contacting respondents, especially former respondents who might no longer identify as polyamorous. In the emails I would mention a research study the person had participated in that was associated with a specific university, but nothing regarding the content of that research.

16. The second university renewed my IRB certification with far more lenient bookkeeping requirements that allowed me to conduct the longitudinal study, but it remained reluctant to grant me permission to talk to children under eighteen years old in poly families. After two additional years of constant revision and reapplication, the IRB summoned me (and my department chair at the time) before the entire board to justify my request to interview children. After yet more revisions and stipulations that one board member privately confided in me seemed "truly insane," the IRB allowed me to finally talk to children in poly families.

3. POLYAMOROUS COMMUNITIES IN THE UNITED STATES

1. (Hutchins 2001: 72)
2. (Muncy 1973: 160)
3. (Muncy 1973: 168)
4. (Hutchins 2001: 72)
5. (Hutchins 2001: 72)
6. (Weeks 1985)
7. (Bornstein 1994; Butler 1990)
8. (Udis-Kessler 1996)
9. (D'Emilio 1983; Weeks 1985)
10. (Stinnet and Birdsong 1978: 104)
11. (Stinnet and Birdsong 1978: 107)
12. (Buunk and van Driel 1989: 134)
13. (Anapol 1997: 97); see also (Francoeur and Francoeur 1974)
14. (Hutchins 2001: 82)
15. (Strassberg 2003: 457)
16. Nearing, personal communication, 2003
17. (Constantine and Constantine 1973: 49)
18. (Smith and Smith 1974)
19. (Smith and Smith 1974)
20. (Bartell 1970)
21. (Bernard 1972)
22. (Ellis 1970)
23. (Bartell 1971; Breedlove and Breedlove 1964; Denfield and Gordon 1970; Fang 1976; Henshel 1973)
24. (Bartell 1970; Jenks 1985)
25. (Flanigan and Zingale 1991)
26. (Gilmartin 1974; Jenks 1985; Levitt 1988)

27. (Bartell 1970; Jenks 1986a)

28. (Jenks 1998: 507)

29. Robert Heinlein, *Stranger in a Strange Land* (New York: Ace, 1987).

30. (Bargh and McKenna 2004; Jenks 1998; Wellman et al. 1996)

31. (Bargh and McKenna 2004)

32. Sex positivity is an outlook that defines sexuality as a positive, life-affirming activity. Proponents define themselves in opposition to "sex negative" Victorian or repressive sexual mores, which cast sexuality as dirty, degrading, or negative.

33. This was not the case when polyamorous groups migrated together to a rural area to establish communities.

34. (Sproull and Faraj 1995)

35. Robert Heinlein's 1961 novel *Stranger in a Strange Land* was especially influential for many people who read its story of nonmonogamous relationships and envisioned creating them in their own lives.

36. (Weinberg et al. 1995: 217)

37. (Weeks, Heaphy, & Donovan 2001: 90)

38. (Weeks, Heaphy, & Donovan 2001)

39. See the Associated Press article on the Divilbliss case at http://www.polyamorysociety.org/Yahoo-Divilbliss_Article.html.

40. http://www.polyamorysociety.org/Divilbiss_Families.html

41. http://www.polyamorysociety.org/Divilbiss_Families_Case_Ends.html

42. http://www.lovemore.com/april/april_divilbiss_case.htm

43. (Durkheim 1960 [1893])

44. (Goffman 1963)

45. Please see http://caw.org/content/?q=bouquet.

46. (Anapol 2012)

47. An exception to the rule, the poly/mono relationship revolves around an explicit agreement allowing both partners equal access to outside lovers, but one chooses to remain monogamous. The monogamous partner often explains his or her abstinence from other partners through her or his monogamous relational orientation.

48. (Merton & Rossi 1968)

49. (Kitsuse 1962; Sartre 1969)

50. A popular read among second-wave polyamorists, see Robert Rimmer, *The Harrad Experiment* (New York: Prometheus Books, 1966).

51. (Spreitzer 2004)

52. (Blanton 1996)

53. See http://www.cnvc.org/ for more information on Nonviolent Communication.

54. (Anapol 2012)

55. (Heinlein 1961)
56. (Rimmer 1966)
57. Ortmann & Sprott 2013)
58. (Bartell 1970; Jenks 1985)
59. (Gilmartin 1974; Jenks 1985; Levitt 1988)
60. (Jenks 1985; Levitt 1988)
61. (Gould 2000; Jenks 1998)
62. (Gould 2000)
63. (Jenks 2001: 171)
64. (Henshel 1973)
65. (Gould 2000)
66. (Bartell 1970; Jenks 1986b)
67. (Gould 2000)
68. (Rust 1993: 368)
69. (Connell 1992 and 2005; Weeks, Heaphy, & Donovan 2001)
70. http://www.poly-nyc.com

4. ISSUES FACING POLY RELATIONSHIPS

1. (Adler and Adler 1987)
2. (Connell 1987 and 2005)
3. (Jenks 1986a; Gould 2000)
4. (Collins 1992; Guttentag and Secord 1983)
5. (Fox 1987: 341); see also (Adler 1985; Henslin 1972)
6. (Adler and Adler 1987: 39)
7. (Adler and Adler 1987: 67)
8. I am not challenging the need for Institutional Research Boards or the validity of what they do. While Institutional Research Boards were created in response to a direct need and they serve a vital function of protecting "human subjects" from potential harms associated with academic research, their sex negativity and legal paranoia has severely impeded me and other sex researchers who have similarly faced outlandish restrictions from which people studying more conventional topics have been exempt.
9. This statement is based on my informal conversations with peers in which I would ask them about the reviews they received from journals and the kinds of documentation the journals required them to produce. Generally, their reviews had a decidedly less personal tone, and none of them had ever been asked to furnish evidence of IRB approval. In contrast, my reviews were personally scathing to a noticeably larger degree than were my colleagues', and

several journals requested evidence of IRB approval when considering my submissions.

10. (Rubin 1992: 150). See also Michel Foucault, *The History of Sexuality* (New York: Vintage, 1990) and Jeffery Weeks, *Sex, Politics, and Society* (Essex, UK: Longman Group, 1981).

11. (Laumann, Gagnon, Michael, & Michaels 1994)

5. CHILDREN IN POLY FAMILIES

1. (Pallotta-Chiarolli 2010)

2. (Constantine & Constantine 1973)

3. A Spanish term meaning mixed or messy, Latina feminists such as Gloria Anzaldua (1987) and Cherrie Moraga (1981) used the term *mestizaje* to describe the multiplistic intersecting natures of sexuality, racial and ethnic identity, gender, religion, politics, and culture. The metaphors of the borderlands, slipping through the cracks between cultures, and mixing disparate elements to become an amalgam that challenges a simplistic bifurcated or dualistic reality are central to the concept of the mestizaje.

4. (Pallotta-Chiarolli 2010: 26)

5. (Pallotta-Chiarolli 2010: 214)

6. In the United States films are rated G for general audiences including small children; PG for parental guidance suggested for small children; PG-13, which is not recommended for children under thirteen; R, which is restricted to anyone under eighteen years old who is not accompanied by an adult; NC-17, which means that no one under eighteen is allowed entrance into the movie; and X, which is pornographic. By saying that the action was PG, Nolan meant that it was very tame and shocking or inappropriate only to very small children or extremely modest people.

7. *Will and Grace* was a popular television show that aired in the United States during the late 1990s and early 2000s and prominently featured several gay characters.

8. (Burde 2013)

6. ADULTS IN POLY FAMILIES

1. See Maria Pallotta-Chiarolli, *Border Sexualities, Border Families in Schools* (Lanham, MD: Rowman & Littlefield, 2010) for more discussion of

her respondents, who also attempted to appear to be perfect to forestall any potential criticism by seeming to be above reproach.

   2. (Baptist and Allen 2008)

   3. (Goldberg 2010)

   4. (Aviram 2007)

   5. (Sheff and Hammers 2011)

   6. (Christensen 1996–1997)

   7. (Adam 2003)

   8. (Card 2007; Emens 2004; Polikoff 1993)

   9. (Sheff 2011)

  10. (Fagan 1999)

  11. W. Rubenstein, "We Are Family: A Reflection on the Search for Legal Recognition of Lesbian and Gay Relationships," *Journal of Law & Politics* 8, no. 89 (1991).

  12. The Society for Creative Anachronism is an "international organization dedicated to researching and recreating the arts and skills of pre-17th century Europe" that hosts gatherings across the United States, http://www.sca.org/, accessed October 24, 2012.

  13. (Ritchie and Barker 2006)

  14. (Weston 1991)

7. BENEFITS OF POLYAMOROUS FAMILY LIFE

   1. (Sheff 2005)

   2. http://officialponyexpress.org/pony-express-quick-facts.html, accessed April 29, 2013.

   3. (Riggs 2010)

   4. See the foundational *Families We Choose: Lesbians, Gays, Kinship* by Kath Weston (1991), as well as *No Place Like Home: Relationships and Family Life among Lesbians and Gay Men* by Christopher Carrington (1999) or *Same Sex Intimacies: Families of Choice and Other Life Experiments* by Jeffrey Weeks, Brian Heaphy, and Catherine Donovan (2001).

   5. (LaRossa 1997)

   6. (Collins 2000; James 1993: 47)

   7. (Collins 2000); See also Wanda Thomas Bernard and Candace Bernard, "Passing the Torch. A Mother and Daughter Reflect on Experiences Across Generations," *Canadian Women's Studies les cahiers de la femme* 18, nos. 2, 3 (Summer/Fall): 46–50.

   8. (Collins 2000)

9. (Mather 2010)

10. (Connell 2005). See also Sheff 2006 for more information on polyhegemonic masculinity.

11. Ibid.

8. DIFFICULTIES IN
POLYAMOROUS FAMILIES

1. (Goffman 1963)

2. (Barker 2005; Califia 2000)

3. (Keres 1994; Wright 2006)

4. (Dalton 2001; Hequembourg 2007; Klein and Moser 2006; Ridinger
2002)

5. (Attias 2004; White 2006)

9. OVERCOMING OBSTACLES

1. (Johnson 2008)

2. (Associated Press April 23, 2003; Kurtz 2003a, 2003b; Lithwick 2004)

3. (Pallotta-Chiarolli 2010: 26)

4. (Pallotta-Chiarolli 2010)

CONCLUSION

1. (Anderlini-D'Onofrio 2005; Bergstrand & Sinski 2010; Rubin 2001)

2. (Kurtz 2003a, 2003b); Stanley Kurtz, "Here Come the Brides : Plural
Marriage Is Waiting in the Wings," *Weekly Standard* 11, no. 15 (December 26,
2005); (Lithwick 2004)

3. (Goldfeder and Sheff 2013)

4. Stephanie Coontz, *Marriage, a History: From Obedience to Intimacy, or
How Love Conquered Marriage* (New York: Viking, 2005).

5. Stephanie Coontz, *The Way We Really Are: Coming to Terms with
America's Changing Families* (New York: Basic Books, 1997).

6. Stephanie Coontz, *The Way We Never Were: American Families and
the Nostalgia Trap* (New York: Basic Books, 1992; new edition with new introduction, 2000).

7. Foundational to this genre is Gayle Rubin's 1984 "Thinking Sex: Notes for a Radical Theory of the Politics of Sexuality," in Carole Vance, ed., *Pleasure and Danger: Exploring Female Sexuality* (New York: Routledge & Kegan Paul). See also the more recent S. Lee, *Erotic Revolutionaries: Black Women, Sexuality, and Popular Culture* (Lanham, MD: Hamilton Books, 2010).

8. (Fonagy et al. 1994)

9. The reality television show *Sister Wives*, aired on TLC, chronicles the lives of the polygynist Fundamentalist Latter-Day Saints (FLDS, also called Fundamentalist Mormons) Brown family with a husband, four wives, and many children as they attempt to navigate life in the contemporary Western United States.

10. (Levine & Silk 1997)

11. (Popenoe 1996)

12. (Cherlin 2010: 405)

13. (Muraco 2006; Oswald 2000, 2002; Weston 1991)

14. (Laumann et al. 1994)

15. (Sheff 2011)

16. In some cases, lesbian couples choose to have the egg of one partner extracted, fertilized, and implanted in the other partner, so both women and the man who provided the sperm are biologically related to the child. Specialized cases like that allow for multiple parentage, but the vast majority of localities allow only two legal parents at any point.

BIBLIOGRAPHY

Adam, B. 2003. "The Defense of Marriage Act and American Exceptionalism: The 'Gay Marriage' Panic in the United States." *Journal of the History of Sexuality* 12, no. 2: 259–76.

Adler, P. 1985. *Wheeling and Dealing.* New York: Columbia University Press.

Adler, P., and Adler, P. 1987. *Membership Roles in Field Research.* Newbury Park: Sage.

Amato, P. 2001. "Children of Divorce in the 1990s: An Update of the Amato and Keith (1991) Meta-Analysis." *Journal of Family Psychology* 15, no. 3: 355–70.

Anapol, D. 1997. *Polyamory, The New Love without Limits: Secrets of Sustainable Intimate Relationships.* San Rafael, CA: IntiNet Resource Center.

———. 2012. *Polyamory in the 21 st Century: Love and Intimacy with Multiple Partners.* Lanham, MD: Rowman & Littlefield.

Anderlini-D'Onofrio, S. 2005. *Plural Loves: Designs for Bi and Poly Living.* New York: Routledge.

Anzaldua, G. 1987. *Borderlands/La Frontera: The New Mestiza.* San Francisco: Spinsters/ Aunt Lute.

Associated Press. 2003. Excerpt from Santorum interview, posted April 23, 2003. Retrieved June 16, 2009. http://www.usatoday.com/news/washington/2003-04-23-santorum-excerpt_x.htm.

Attias, B. 2004. "'Police Free Gay Slaves': Consent, Sexuality, and the Law." *Left History* 10, no. 1: 55–83.

Aviram, Hadar. 2007. "Make Love, Not Law: Perceptions of the Marriage Equality Struggle among Polyamorous Activists." *Journal of Bisexuality* 7, no. 3–4: 263–86.

Baptist, J., and Allen, K. 2008. "A Family's Coming Out Process: Systemic Change and Multiple Realities." *Contemporary Family Therapy* 30: 92–110.

Bargh, J., and McKenna, K. 2004. "The Internet and Social Life." *Annual Review of Psychology* 55: 573–90.

Barker, M. 2005. "On Tops, Bottoms and Ethical Sluts: The Place of BDSM and Polyamory in Lesbian and Gay Psychology." *Lesbian and Gay Psychology Review* 6, no. 2: 124–29.

Bartell, G. 1970. "Group Sex Among the Mid-Americans." *Journal of Sex Research* 6, no. 2: 113–30.

———. 1971. *Group Sex: A Scientist's Eyewitness Report on the American Way of Swinging.* New York: Van Rees Press.

Baxter, J., Hewitt, B., and Western, M. 2005. "Post-Familial Families and the Domestic Division of Labour." *Journal of Comparative Family Studies*: 583–600.

Bergstrand, C., and Sinski, J. 2010. *Swinging in America: Love, Sex, and Marriage in the 21st Century.* New York: Praeger.

Bernard, Jessie. 1972. *The Future of Marriage*. New Haven: Yale University Press.

Bernard, Wanda, and Bernard, Candace. 1998. "Passing the Torch. A Mother and Daughter Reflect on Experiences Across Generations." *Canadian Women's Studies les cahiers de la femme* 18, no. 2, 3 (Summer/Fall): 46–50.

Bettinger, M. 2005. "Polyamory and Gay Men: A Family Systems Approach." *Journal of GLBT Family Studies* 1, no. 1: 97–116.

Blanton, B. 1996. *Radical Honesty*. New York: Dell Publishing.

Block, J. 2008. *Open: Love, Sex, and Life in an Open Marriage*. Berkeley, CA: Seal Press.

Bornstein, K. 1994. *Gender Outlaw: On Men, Women, and the Rest of Us*. New York: Routledge.

Breedlove, W., and Breedlove, J. 1964. *Swap Clubs: A Study in Contemporary Sexual Mores*. Los Angeles: Sherbourne Press.

Bumpass, L., and Raley, R. 1995. "Redefining Single-Parent Families: Cohabitation and Changing Family Reality." *Demography* 32, no. 1: 97–109.

Burde, Jessica. 2013. *The Polyamory on Purpose Guide to Polyamory and Pregnancy*. Memphis, TN: Self-published.

Butler, J. 1990. *Gender Trouble: Feminism and the Subversion of Identity*. London: Routledge.

Buunk, Abraham P., and van Driel, B. 1989. *Variant Lifestyles and Relationships*. London: Sage Publications, Ltd.

Califia, P. 2000. *Public Sex: The Culture of Radical Sex*. San Francisco: Cleis Press.

Card, Claudia. 2007. "Gay Divorce: Thoughts on the Legal Regulation of Marriage." *Hypatia* 22, no. 1: 24–38.

Carrington, Christopher. 1999. *No Place Like Home: Relationships and Family Life among Lesbians and Gay Men*. Chicago, IL: The University of Chicago Press.

Cherlin, Andrew. 2010. "Demographic Trends in the United States: A Review of Research in the 2000s." *Journal of Marriage and Family* 72: 403–19.

Christensen, C. 1996–1997. "Legal Ordering of Family Values: The Case of Gay and Lesbian Families." *Cardozo Law Review*: 1299–1352.

Collins, P. H. 1992. "Transforming the Inner Circle: Dorothy Smith's Challenge to Sociological Theory." *Sociological Theory* 10, no. 1 (Spring): 73–80.

———. 2000. *Black Feminist Thought: Knowledge, Consciousness, and Politics of Empowerment*. New York: Psychology Press.

Connell, R. W. 1987. *Gender and Power: Society, the Person, and Sexual Politics*. Sydney: Allen and Unwin.

———. 1992. "A Very Straight Gay: Masculinity, Homosexual Experience, and the Dynamics of Gender." *American Sociological Review* 7, no. 6 (December): 735–51.

———. 2005. *Masculinities* (Second Edition). Los Angeles: University of California Press.

Constantine, L., and Constantine, J. 1973. *Group Marriage: A Study of Contemporary Multilateral Marriage*. New York: Collier Books.

Coontz, Stephanie. 1988. *Social Origins of Private Life: A History of American Families 1600–1900*. New York: Verso.

———. 1992. *The Way We Never Were: American Families and the Nostalgia Trap*. New York: Basic Books.

———. 1998. *The Way We Really Are: Coming to Terms with America's Changing Families*. New York: Basic Books.

———. 2005. *Marriage, A History: From Obedience to Intimacy, or How Love Conquered Marriage*. New York: Viking.

Dalton, Susan. 2001. "Protecting Our Parent-Child Relationships: Understanding the Strengths and Weaknesses of Second-Parent Adoption." In *Queer Families, Queer Politics: Challenging Culture and the State*, edited by Mary Bernstein and Renate Reimann, 201–20. New York: Columbia University Press.

D'Emilio, J. 1983. *Sexual Politics, Sexual Communities: The Making of a Homosexual Minority in the United States, 1940–1970*. Chicago: University of Chicago Press.

Denfeld, D., and Gordon, M. 1970. "The Sociology of Mate Swapping: or The Family That Swings Together Clings Together." *Journal of Sex Research* 6, no. 2: 85–100.

Durkheim, Emile. 1960 [1893]. *The Division of Labor in Society*. Translated by George Simpson. New York: The Free Press.

Easton, Dossie, and Liszt, Catherine A. 1997. *The Ethical Slut: A Guide to Infinite Possibilities*. San Francisco: Greenery Press.

Edin, K., and Kefalas, M. 2005. *Promises I Can Keep: Why Low-Income Women Put Motherhood before Marriage*. University of California Press.

Ellis, A. 1970. "Group Marriage: A Possible Alternative?" In *The Family in Search of a Future*, edited by H. Otto. New York: Appleton-Century-Crofts.

Emens, Elizabeth. 2004. "Monogamy's Law: Compulsory Monogamy and Polyamorous Existence." *New York University Review of Law and Social Change* 29: 277.

Fagan, P. F. (1999). How broken families rob children of their chances for future prosperity. *Backgrounder*, (1283).

Fang, B. 1976. "Swinging: In Retrospect." *The Journal of Sex Research* 12 (August).

Flanigan, W., and Zingale, N. 1991. *Political Behavior of the American Electorate* (seventh edition). Washington DC: CQ Press.

Fonagy, P., Steele, M., Steele, H., Higgitt, A., and Target, M. 1994. "The Emanuel Miller Memorial Lecture 1992: The Theory and Practice of Resilience." *Journal of Child Psychology and Psychiatry* 35, no. 2: 231–57.

Foucault, Michel. 1978. *The History of Sexuality, Vol. 1: An Introduction*. Harmondsworth: Penguin.

Fox, K. 1987. "Real Punks and Pretenders: The Social Organization of a Counterculture." *Journal of Contemporary Ethnography* 16, no. 3.

Francoeur, A., and Francoeur, R. 1974. *Hot and Cool Sex: Cultures in Conflict*. New York: Harcourt, Brace, and Jovanovich.

Gilmartin, B. 1974. "Sexual Deviance and Social Networks: A Study of Social, Family, and Marital Interaction Patterns among Co-marital Sex Participants." In *Beyond Monogamy: Recent Studies of Sexual Alternatives in Marriage*, edited by J. R. Smith and L. G. Smith. Baltimore: Johns Hopkins Press.

Goffman, Erving. 1963. *Stigma: Notes on the Management of Spoiled Identity*. New York: Touchstone, Simon and Shuster.

Goldberg, Abbie. 2010. *Lesbian and Gay Parents and Their Children: Research on the Family Life Cycle*. Washington, DC: The American Psychological Association.

Goldfeder, Mark and Sheff, Elisabeth. 2013. "Children in Polyamorous Families: A First Empirical Look," *The Journal of Law and Social Deviance*. Volume 5, pages 150–243. http://www.lsd-journal.net/archives/Volume5/ChildrenOfPolyamorousFamilies.pdf

Gould, Terry. 2000. *The Lifestyle: A Look at the Erotic Rites of Swingers*. Vintage Canada.

Guttentag, M., and Secord, P. 1983. *Too Many Women? The Sex Ratio Question*. London: Sage.

Heinlein, R. 1961. *Stranger in a Strange Land*. New York: Ace.

Henshel, A. 1973. "Swinging: A Study of Decision Making in Marriage." *American Journal of Sociology* 78, no. 4: 885–91.

Henslin, J. 1972. "Studying Deviance in Four Settings: Research Experiences with Cabbies, Suicides, Drug Users, and Abortionees." In *Research on Deviance*, edited by J. Douglas. New York: Random House.

Hequembourg, A. 2007. *Lesbian Motherhood: Stories of Becoming*. Routledge: New York.

Hetherington, E. M., and Stanley-Hagan, M. 1999. "The Adjustment of Children with Divorced Parents: A Risk and Resiliency Perspective." *Journal of Child Psychology and Psychiatry* 40, no. 1: 129–40.

Hutchins, Loraine. 2001. *Erotic Rites: A Cultural Analysis of Contemporary US Sacred Sexuality Traditions and Trends*. Unpublished dissertation for the Cultural Studies Department, Union Institute Graduate College.

James, Stanlie M. 1993. "Mothering: A Possible Black Feminist Link to Social Transformation." In *Theorizing Black Feminisms: The Visionary Pragmatism of Black Women*, edited by Stanlie M. James and Abena P. A. Busia. London: Routledge.

Jenks, R. 1985. "A Comparative Study of Swingers and Non-Swingers: Attitudes and Beliefs." *Lifestyles: Journal of Changing Patterns* 7: 5–20.

————. 1986a. "Swinging: A Test of Two Theories and a Proposed New Model." *Archives of Sexual Behavior* 14, no. 6: 517–27.

————. 1986b. "Swinging: A Review of the Literature." *Archives of Sexual Behavior* 27, no. 5: 507–22.

————. 1998. "Swinging: A Review of the Literature." *Archives of Sexual Behavior* 27, no. 5: 507–21.

————. 2001. *"The Lifestyle: A Look at the Erotic Rites of Swingers, by Terry Gould." Journal of Sex Research* 38, no. 2: 171–73.

Johnson, M. 2008. *A Typology of Domestic Violence: Intimate Terrorism, Violent Resistance, and Situational Couple Violence.* Boston: University Press of New England.

Keres, J. 1994. "Violence against S/M Women within the Lesbian Community: A Nation-Wide Survey." *Female Trouble.* National Coalition for Sexual Freedom, downloaded November 5, 2009, https://ncsfreedom.org/component/k2/item/453-violence-against-s/m-women-within-the-lesbian-community-a-nation-wide-survey.html.

Kitsuse, J. 1962. "Societal Reactions to Deviant Behavior: Problems of Theory and Method." *Social Problems* 9: 247–56.

Klein, M. and Moser, C. 2006. "SM (Sadomasochistic) Interests in a Child Custody Proceeding." *Journal of Homosexuality* 50.

Kurtz, S. 2003a. "Heather Has 3 Parents." *National Review Online*, March 12. Retrieved September 12, 2006, http://www.nationalreview.com/articles/206153/heather-has-3-parents/stanley-kurtz.

————. 2003b. "Beyond Gay Marriage." *The Weekly Standard* 8, no. 45 (August 4–11), http://www.weeklystandard.com/Content/Public/Articles/000/000/002/938xpsxy.asp.

LaRossa, R. 1997. *The Modernization of Fatherhood: A Social and Political History.* Chicago: University of Chicago Press.

Laumann, E., Gagnon, J., Michael, R., and Michaels, S. 1994. *The Social Organization of Sexuality.* Chicago: University of Chicago Press.

Lee, S. 2010. *Erotic Revolutionaries: Black Women, Sexuality, and Popular Culture.* Lanham, MD: Hamilton Books.

Levine, Nancy, and Silk, Joan. 1997. "Why Polyandry Fails: Sources of Instability in Polyandrous Marriages." *Current Anthropology* 38, no. 3: 375–98.

Levitt, E. 1988. "Alternative Life Style and Marital Satisfaction." *Annals of Sex Research* 1: 455–61.

Lithwick, D. 2004. Slippery Slop. *Slate*, May 19, 2004. Retrieved June 2, 2009, http://www.slate.com/id/2100824/.

Madow, M., and Hardy, S. 2010. "Incidence and Analysis of the Broken Family in the Background of Neurosis." *American Journal of Orthopsychiatry* 17, no. 3: 521–28.

Mather, M. 2010. "U.S. Children in Single-Mother Families." *Population Reference Bureau*, Washington, D.C. http://www.prb.org/pdf10/single-motherfamilies.pdf. Accessed July 28, 2013.

McCubbin, H., and McCubbin, M. 1988. "Typologies of Resilient Families: Emerging Roles of Social Class and Ethnicity." *Family Relations* 37, no. 3: 247–54.

Merton, R., and Rossi, A. 1968. "Contributions to the Theory of Reference Group Behavior." In *Social Theory and Social Structure*, edited by Robert Merton. New York: Free Press.

Moraga, C. 1981. "The Welder." In *This Bridge Called My Back: Writings of Radical Women of Color*, edited by C. Moraga and G. Anzaldua. Watertown, MA: Persephone Press.

Muncy, R. 1973. *Sex and Marriage in Utopian Communities.* Bloomington, IA: Indiana University Press.

Muraco, A. 2006. "Intentional Families: Fictive Kin Ties between Cross-Gender, Different Sexual Orientation Friends." *Journal of Marriage and Family* 68: 1313–25.

Nearing, R. (ed.). 1992. *Loving More: The Polyfidelity Primer.* Honolulu, HI: Pep Publishing.

Olsson, C., Bond, L., Burns, J., Vella-Brodick, D., and Sawyer, S. 2003. "Adolescent Resilience: A Concept Analysis." *Journal of Adolescence* 26: 1–11.

Ortmann, D., and Sprott, R. 2013. *Sexual Outsiders: Understanding BDSM Sexualities and Communities.* Lanham, MD: Rowman and Littlefield.

Oswald, R. 2000. "A Member of the Wedding? Heterosexism and Family Ritual." *Journal of Social and Personal Relationships* 17, no. 3: 349–68.
———. 2002. "Resilience within the Family Networks of Lesbians and Gay Men: Intentionality and Redefinition." *Journal of Marriage and Family* 64, no. 2: 374–84.
Pallotta-Chiarolli, M. 2006. "Polyparents Having Children, Raising Children, Schooling Children." *Lesbian and Gay Psychology Review* 7, no. 1: 48–53.
———. 2010a. *Border Sexualities, Border Families in Schools.* Lanham, MD: Rowman & Littlefield.
———. 2010b. "To Pass, Border, or Pollute: Polyfamilies Go to School." In M. Barker and D. Langdridge, *Understanding Non-Monogamies,* 182–87. New York: Routledge.
Pallotta-Chiarolli, M., and Lubowitz, S. 2003. "Outside Belonging: Multi-Sexual Relationships as Border Existence." *Journal of Bisexuality* 3, no. 1: 53–86.
Patterson, J. 2002. "Understanding Family Resilience." *Journal of Clinical Psychology* 58, no. 3: 233–46.
Polikoff, N. 1993. "We Will Get What We Ask For: Why Legalizing Gay and Lesbian Marriage Will Not Dismantle the Legal Structure of Gender in Every Marriage." *Virginia Law Review* 79, no. 7: 1535–50.
———. 2008. *Beyond (Straight and Gay) Marriage: Valuing All Families under the Law.* Boston: Beacon Press.
Popenoe, D. 1996. *Life without Father.* New York: Free Press.
Ridinger, R. 2002. "Things Visible and Invisible: The Leather Archives and Museum." *Journal of Homosexuality* 43: 1–9.
Riggs, D. 2010. "Developing a 'Responsible' Foster Care Praxis: Poly as a Framework for Examining Power and Propriety in Family Contexts." In *Understanding Non-Monogamies,* edited by M. Barker and D. Langdridge. London: Routledge.
Rimmer, R. 1966. *The Harrad Experiment.* New York: Prometheus Books.
Ritchie, A., and Barker, M. 2006. "'There Aren't Words for What We Do or How We Feel So We Have to Make Them Up': Constructing Polyamorous Languages in a Culture of Compulsory Monogamy." *Sexualities* 9, no. 5: 584–601.
Rubin, G. 1992. "Thinking Sex: Notes for a Radical Theory of the Politics of Sexuality." In *Culture, Society, and Sexuality: A Reader,* 150. Edited by Peter Aggleton and Richard Parke. UCL Press: London.
Rubin, R. 2001. "Alternative Family Lifestyles Revisited, or Whatever Happened to Swingers, Group Marriages and Communes?" *Journal of Family Issues* 7, no. 6: 711–27.
Rust, P. 1993. "Coming Out in the Age of Social Constructionism: Sexual Identity Formation among Lesbian and Bisexual Women." *Gender & Society* 7, no. 1: 711–27.
———. 2000. "Bisexuality: A Contemporary Paradox for Women." *Journal of Social Issues* 56: 205–21.
——— 2003. "Monogamy and Polyamory: Relationship Issues for Bisexuals." In *Psychological Perspectives on Lesbian, Gay, and Bisexual Experiences* (second edition), edited by Linda D. Garnets and Douglas C. Kimmel, 475–96. New York: Columbia University Press.
Sartre, J. 1969. *The Wall: Intimacy.* New York: New Directions Publishing.
Sheff, E. 2005a. "Polyamorous Women, Sexual Subjectivity, and Power." *Journal of Contemporary Ethnography* 34, no. 3: 251–83.
———. 2005b. *Gender, Family, and Sexuality: Exploring Polyamorous Community.* Unpublished doctoral dissertation submitted to the Faculty of the Graduate School of the University of Colorado in partial fulfillment of the requirement for the degree of Doctor of Philosophy, Department of Sociology.
———. 2006. "Poly-Hegemonic Masculinities." *Sexualities* 9, no. 5: 621–42.
———. 2007. "The Reluctant Polyamorist: Auto-Ethnographic Research in a Sexualized Setting." In *Sex Matters: The Sexuality and Society Reader* (second edition), edited by M. Stombler, D. Baunach, E. Burgess, D. Donnelly, and W. Simonds, 111–18. New York: Pearson, Allyn, and Bacon.
———. 2011. "Polyamorous Families, Same-Sex Marriage, and the Slippery Slope." *Journal of Contemporary Ethnography* 40, no. 5: 487–520.

Sheff, E., and Hammers, C. 2011. "The Privilege of Perversities: Race, Class, and Education Among Polyamorists and Kinksters." *Sexuality & Psychology* 2, no. 3: 198–223.

Skolnik, A. 1991. *Embattled Paradise: The American Family in an Age of Uncertainty.* New York: Basic Books.

Smith, D. 1974. "Women's Perspective as a Radical Critique of Sociology." *Sociological Inquiry* 44: 7–13.

Smith, J. and Smith, L. (eds.). 1974. *Beyond Monogamy: Recent Studies of Sexual Alternatives in Marriage.* Baltimore: The Johns Hopkins University Press.

Spanier, G., and Cole, C. 1975. "Mate Swapping: Perceptions, Value Orientations, and Participation in a Midwestern Community." *Archives of Sexual Behavior* 4, no. 2: 143–59.

Spreitzer, G. 2004. "Toward the Construct Definition of Positive Deviance." *American Behavioral Scientist* 47, no. 6 (February): 828–47.

Sproull, L. and Faraj, S. 1995. "Atheism, Sex and Databases: The Net as a Social Technology." In *Public Access to the Internet*, edited by B. Kahin and J. Keller. Cambridge: MIT Press.

Stacey, J. 1996. *In the Name of the Family: Rethinking Family Values in the Postmodern Age.* Boston: Beacon Press.

———. 2003. "Gay and Lesbian Families: Queer Like Us." In *All Our Families: New Policies for a New Century*, edited by Mary Mason, Arlene Skolnik, and Stephen Sugarman. New York: Oxford University Press.

Stinnett, N. and Birdsong, C. 1978. *The Family and Alternate Lifestyles.* Chicago: Nelson-Hall.

Strassberg, M. 2003. "The Challenge of Post-Modern Polygamy: Considering Polyamory." *Capital University Law Review* 31, no. 3: 439–563.

Sullivan, M. 2004. *The Family of Woman: Lesbian Mothers, Their Children, and the Undoing of Gender.* Berkeley, CA: University of California Press.

Udis-Kessler, A. 1996. "Identity/Politics: Historical Sources of the Bisexual Movement." In *Queer Studies: A Lesbian, Gay, Bisexual, and Transgender Anthology.* New York: New York University Press.

Waite, L. and Gallagher, M. 2000. *The Case for Marriage: Why Married People Are Happier, Healthier, and Better Off Financially.* New York: Doubleday.

Walsh, F. 2002. "A Family Resilience Framework: Innovative Practice Applications." *Family Relations* 51, no. 2: 130–37.

Weeks, J. 1985. *Sexuality and Its Discontents: Meanings, Myths, and Modern Sexualities.* London: Routledge, Kegan and Paul.

Weeks, J., Heaphy, B., and Donovan, C. 2001. *Same Sex Intimacies: Families of Choice and Other Life Experiments.* London: Routledge, Kegan, and Paul.

Weinberg, M., Williams, C., and Calhan, C. 1995. "'If the Shoe Fits' . . . : Exploring Male Homosexual Foot Fetishism." *Journal of Sex Research* 32, no. 1: 17–27.

Wellman, B. and Gulia, M. 1995. "Net Surfers Don't Ride Alone: Virtual Communities as Communities." Paper presented at the American Sociological Association session on "Reinventing Community," Washington, D.C.

Wellman, B., Salaff, J., Dimitrova, D., Garton, L., Gulia, M., and Haythornthwaite, C. 1996. "Computer Networks as Social Networks: Collaborative Work, Telework, and Virtual Community." *Annual Review of Sociology* 22: 213–38.

Weston, K. 1991. *Families We Choose: Lesbians, Gays, Kinship.* New York: Columbia University Press.

White, C. 2006. "The Spanner Trials and Changing Laws on Sadomasochism in the UK." In *Sadomasochism: Powerful Pleasures*, edited by P. Kleinplatz and C. Moser. New York: Hayworth Press.

Wilson, J. 2002. *The Marriage Problem: How Our Culture Has Weakened Families.* New York: Harper Collins.

Wright, S. 2006. "Discrimination of SM-Identified Individuals." *Journal of Homosexuality* 50, no. 2: 217–31.

Yip, A. 1997. "Gay Male Christian Couples and Sexual Exclusivity." *Sociologu* 31, no. 2: 289–306.

INDEX

Activism, poly *see also* Poly Pride Day NYC: Being out as activist, 226

Age *see also* children, polygeezers, teens: Adult children reject poly parent, 219–223; Age-appropriate answers, importance of, 191–192; Influence on makeup of poly communities, 27; Older people, Polygeezers, 27; Teens, 139–140; Tweens, 137–139; Very young children missing from the sample, 38; Young children, 136–137; Young people and hookup culture, 27

Autonomy: As element of choice, 24; As source of power, 28; Primary relationship with self, 19

Benefits of poly family life *see also* autonomy, children, chosen kinship, community, emotional intimacy, emotional protection, freedom, family poly, honesty, parenting, resources, sexuality: Accommodating disabilities, 198–199; Attention for children, 201–202; Easier coparenting after divorce, 206; Easier to get dates, makes you more interesting, 201; Family expansion, 206–209; Honesty cultivates emotional intimacy, 191–195; More loot, 197; More sleep with new baby, 200; Multiple partners provide protection from Intimate

Partner Violence, 261–262; Parents ability to remain friendly after divorce, 205–206, 212; Role models for children, 203–205; Shared resources, money, 196; Shared resources, parental attention and expertise, 203; Shared resources, time, 199–201; Smooth function of poly family *see also* children comfortable in family, 10, 11, 194–195, 201, 271; Social stimulation, 197, 203, 241

Bisexuality *see also* gay, gender, lesbian, lesbigay, sexual minority: As advantageous to women in poly communities, 29, 88; As entertaining to men, 30, 88; Coffee night in the Bay Area, 88; Invisibility of, 30; Overlap with poly community, 74; Threat of male bisexuality, 30, 86–87, 88

BDSM *see also* kinkster, kinky: Definition of, 38, 73; Differences in desire for, 38–39

Break-up *see also* divorce, relationships: Still friends with polyaffective partner, 211, 212

Celibacy: While married, 26

Change *see also* continuity: Acceptable, not a signal of failure, 185–186, 186, 188, 280; In poly families, 9, 14–15, 178, 188, 274–276, 280–281; Needs